Paediatric Cases in Coloured Skin

Dermatology is a visual discipline in which observation to detail is key to accurate diagnosis, especially in children. This book for clinicians provides a clear and easy guide to identify skin diseases in children with coloured skin. It discusses more than 112 skin problems with over 192 colour photographs following a logical organization with picture-based Q&A at the end. It features skin problems specific to children such as haemangiomas, congenital naevi, neurocutaneous syndromes, napkin rash, etc., as well as those also seen in adults such as psoriasis, lichen planus, and eczema. This book also covers tropical diseases such as cutaneous tuberculosis, leishmaniasis, fungal infections, and leprosy.

KEY FEATURES

- Highlights the differences in clinical presentation in children having coloured skin
- Stimulates the interest in tropical dermatology and skin problems in coloured skin, among medical students, trainees, general practitioners, paediatricians, and dermatologists
- Features high-quality colour photographs and concise, practical text for accurate diagnosis and effective treatment

Paediatric Cases
in Coloured Skin

Ranthilaka R. Gammanpila MBBS MD
Department of Dermatology
Teaching Hospital Kalutara, Sri Lanka

Ajith P. Kannangara MBBS MD
Department of Dermatology
Teaching Hospital Kalutara, Sri Lanka

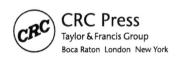

CRC Press
Taylor & Francis Group
Boca Raton London New York

CRC Press is an imprint of the
Taylor & Francis Group, an **informa** business

Designed cover image: Authors

First edition published 2024
by CRC Press
2385 NW Executive Center Drive, Suite 320, Boca Raton FL 33431

and by CRC Press
4 Park Square, Milton Park, Abingdon, Oxon, OX14 4RN

CRC Press is an imprint of Taylor & Francis Group, LLC

© 2024 Ranthilaka R. Gammanpila and Ajith P. Kannangara

ISBN: 978-1-032-34316-7 (hbk)
ISBN: 978-1-032-34315-0 (pbk)
ISBN: 978-1-003-32150-7 (ebk)

DOI: 10.1201/9781003321507

Typeset in Times
by Apex CoVantage, LLC

We authors dedicate this book to those people of Sri Lanka
who are proud of their striking brown skin.

Contents

Preface

Skin lesions are one of the most common human diseases. The diversity of skin colour creates challenges for the objective diagnosis, especially in children. Diagnosis in dermatology is largely based on visual inspection of a lesion or the suspicious skin area. Erythema is inconspicuous and post-inflammatory hypopigmentation and hyperpigmentation is marked in coloured skin children. For example, PASI score in psoriasis is much lower in a darker-skinned child of the same severity due to 0 or 1 erythema score; genital lichen sclerosus presents early as darker-skinned children notice depigmentation early, mistaken for vitiligo; erythematous, oedematous, inflammatory phase, "lilac ring" or yellowish white sclerotic phase described in morphoea in white skin is rarely observed in brown-skinned patients. Therefore, it is important to get familiar with clinical manifestations in different skin colours to minimize mismanagements.

Dermatology training aims to improve the ability of physicians to correctly diagnose a skin lesion, and the efficacy of their education depends largely on the number of images utilized for their training. The most leading text books today overrepresent light skin tone (74.5%) and underrepresent dark skin tone (4.5%), while more than two thirds are skin of colour in the world population. Identifying this necessity, we published our first book on brown skin in 2021: Ranawaka R.R., Kannangara A.P., Karawita A. (eds) *Atlas of Dermatoses in Pigmented Skin* (2021). Springer, Singapore. https://doi.org/10.1007/978-981-15-5483-4_15

The current book is written for medical students, postgraduate trainees, general practitioners, and dermatologists who treat children with brown skin, Fitzpatrick type V. This book discusses *112 skin diseases using 192 colour photographs*. This is a good platform for pharmaceutical industries and scientists to research on optimum topical therapies for different skin colours.

About the Authors

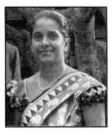

Dr. Ranthilaka R. Gammanpila, MBBS MD, (Ranawaka) is the consultant dermatologist at Teaching Hospital Kalutara, Sri Lanka. She qualified MBBS (1996) and MD (2004) from the University of Colombo and had one year of research training at St. John's Institute of Dermatology in the UK (2006).

She is the editor of the first international medical book published in Sri Lanka: *Atlas of Dermatoses in Pigmented Skin* (2021). Springer, Singapore https://doi.org/10.1007/978-81-15-5483-4_15. She has been the author of 27 chapters in international dermatology books; has published 28 scientific papers in indexed journals including six clinical trials; and has authored 8 medical books nationally. Her main areas of research interest are leishmaniasis, cutaneous tuberculosis, onychomycosis, and leprosy. She was the first Sri Lankan dermatologist to represent her motherland at the World Congress of Dermatology (WCD2019, Milan, Italy) being a co-chair and a guest speaker. Currently, she contributes to international books emphasizing the clinical differences in brown skin versus white skin.

In 2022, she published her first short novel highlighting the whys and wherefores of current economic failure in Sri Lanka in the background of her personal experiences.

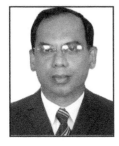

Dr. Ajith P. Kannangara, MBBS MD, consultant dermatologist, specialist in anti-aging medicine and cosmetic dermatology, is currently attached to the Ministry of Health, Teaching Hospital, Karapitiya, Galle, Sri Lanka. He obtained his MBBS from the University of Peradeniya and MD (dermatology) from the University of Colombo, Sri Lanka. Dr. Kannangara received the National Skin Centre and Stiefel Fellowship from the National Skin Centre, Singapore and post-doctoral International Dermatology Fellow from Wake Forest University Baptist Medical Centre, North Carolina, USA. He also obtained a diploma from the American Academy of Anti-Aging and Regenerative Medicine (A4M) and American Academy of Aesthetic Medicine (A3M).

Dr. Kannangara also serves as editor and reviewer for various national and international journals. His research papers are published in most renowned national and international journals of dermatology, and he is among the co-editors of the recently published book *Atlas of Dermatoses in Pigmented Skin*. He is one of the pioneers of the proposed classification of cutaneous reactions (Koebner, Wolf's isotopic, Renbök, Koebner nonreaction, Wolf's isotopic nonreaction, immunocompromised district, and other phenomena), and introduced the concept of the sparing phenomenon.

Dr. Kannangara is the founding and current president of Skin Sri Lanka which is an associate member of the International Alliance of Dermatology Patient Organizations, or GlobalSkin.

Acknowledgements

We acknowledge our patients who are the source of our knowledge and inspiration. Also, we thank the publishers for all their help at every stage of the publication, for their tireless efforts, their constant reminders, and for putting up with us through the editorial process.

Congenital Naevi and Haemangiomas in Children with FST 5

1

Ranthilaka R. Gammanpila

INTRODUCTION

This chapter discusses common congenital naevi and haemangiomas in children with brown skin (Fitzpatrick skin type V/FST 5). These are discussed based on a clinical photograph and easy-to-read question-and-answer format. In fact, the erythema is mild and inconspicuous in darker skin and may lead to fatality if not vigilant. Also, some naevi are more common in darker-skinned children such as blue sacral naevus and hypopigmented naevus. Even though the most clinical descriptions are same for both white and brown skin, the differences we noted are highlighted under each case discussion.

CONGENITAL NAEVI

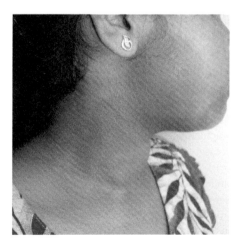

FIGURE 1.1A An 11-year-old girl came with progressively enlarging blackish patch on the face and the neck. That has recently appeared and was not since birth. Note the hypertrichosis on the lesion.

DOI: 10.1201/9781003321507-1

Based on the case description and Figure 1.1a, what are your differential diagnoses?

1. Congenital melanocytic naevus (CMN)
2. Becker naevus

BECKER NAEVUS

Diagnosis

Becker naevus (pigmented hairy epidermal naevus, Becker melanosis)

Discussion

Becker naevus, or pigmented hairy epidermal naevus, is a hamartoma that usually presents with hyperpigmentation affecting the upper back, flanks, or upper chest. It is frequently but not always hypertrichotic, and is commonest on the upper trunk. Incidence is around 0.25%, and is commoner in males than females.

The majority of lesions appear around puberty, then slowly enlarges in the first two decades, then remain the same throughout. When it is associated with extracutaneous abnormalities it is termed Becker naevus syndrome, which can involve underlying structures, namely aplasia or hypoplasia of the underlying breast tissue, or pectoralis major muscle (or sometimes shoulder muscles), or lipoatrophy. Other extracutaneous associations described are ipsilateral limb growth disturbance, supernumerary nipples, and scoliosis (Kinsler & Sebire, 2016, 75.19).

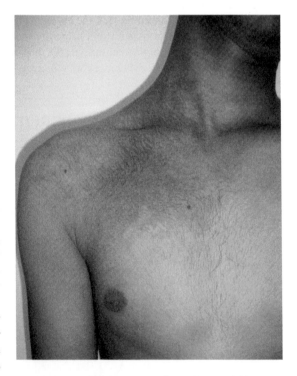

Investigations

This is a clinical diagnosis.

Management

- Pigment-targeting Q-switched lasers, such as the 694-nm Q-switched ruby, 1064-nm Q-switched Nd:YAG, and 755-nm Q-switched alexandrite lasers selectively damage epidermal and dermal melanin without removing the entire epidermis. Many treatment sessions are necessary.
- Fractional Erbium: YAG (2940 nm) laser is a promising new treatment modality for Becker naevus. No adverse effects were observed, and the safety profile appears to be fairly broad (Al-Bakaa, 2022).

FIGURE 1.1B   Becker naevus in a 16-year-old boy.

Based on the case description and Figure 1.2, what are your differential diagnoses?

1. Blue sacral naevus or Mongolian blue spot
2. Congenital melanocytic naevus (CMN)

BLUE SACRAL NAEVUS OR MONGOLIAN BLUE SPOT

Diagnosis

Blue sacral naevus or Mongolian blue spot

Discussion

Mongolian spot is a dermal melanocytic lesion which is formed due to hypermelanosis, in which an increased number of melanocytes are entrapped in the dermis (dermal melanocytosis), causing the bluish grey colour (Tindall effect). They are varying in size and shape located on the sacral area in normal infants. The colour increases in depth for a period during infancy and then diminishes. It has a round or oval shape, with a diameter of usually up to 10 centimetres. Normally it presents as a single lesion, but multiple Mongolian spots may occasionally occur. The most common location is the lumbosacral region. This is more common in darker skin (13–26%) and uncommon in white skin (Gupta, 2013).

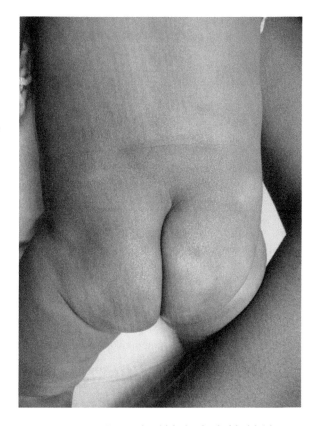

Investigations

This is a clinical diagnosis.

FIGURE 1.2 A 2-month-old baby had this bluish-grey patch on the back of the trunk since birth. The mother wants to know whether this will persist for life.

Management

Mongolian spots typically resolve during childhood; therefore, no treatment is required. Occasionally this may persist into adult life. Persistent cases have been treated with Q-switched lasers, intense pulsed light, and bleaching creams.

Based on the case description and Figure 1.3, what are your differential diagnoses?

1. Linear congenital epidermal naevus
2. Inflammatory linear verrucous epidermal naevus (ILVEN)
3. Linear lichen planus
4. Pigmentary mosaicism

LINEAR CONGENITAL EPIDERMAL NAEVUS

Diagnosis

Linear congenital epidermal naevus (keratinocytic naevus)

Discussion

Congenital epidermal naevi (CEN) present at birth or become apparent in the first years of life. The phenotype can develop over the first years, and often become more pronounced with age, particularly with increasing hyperkeratosis in keratinocytic naevi. Single CEN lesions can be either round or linear, but larger or multiple lesions appear in Blaschko linear distribution.

Epidermal naevi are very superficial and are therefore raised, and can have the appearance of being "stuck on" to the surface of the skin. Their surface characteristics depend on the cell type that predominates. Keratinocytic naevi vary from brown to blackish in FST 5, and nearly macular with a soft velvety feel to verrucous or hyperkeratotic, and can have a prominent inflammatory component (ILVEN).

There are several clearly delineated CEN syndromes: HRAS mosaicism, Proteus syndrome, CHILD syndrome, PENS syndrome, Becker naevus syndrome, follicular naevus/naevus comedonicus syndrome, etc. (Kinsler & Sebire 2016, 75.3, 75.14).

Investigations

This is a clinical diagnosis. Phenotype can be confirmed by histopathology.

Management

CEN are permanent if not surgically removed. Surgical excision can be suitable for small, single, epidermal naevi. Keratinocytic and sebaceous naevi are candidates for ablative laser therapy to reduce thickness and/or hyperkeratosis of the lesion. Smaller verrucous lesions have been treated successfully with cryotherapy. ILVEN have been treated with CO2 laser (Paasch et al., 2022).

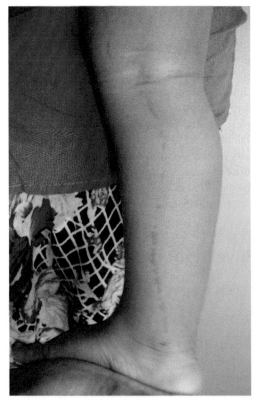

FIGURE 1.3 A 14-month-old baby girl came with this hyperpigmented linear lesion on the right leg. The mother was worried because it rapidly extended along the leg.

Based on the case description and Figure 1.4, what are your differential diagnoses?

1. Congenital melanocytic naevus (CMN)
2. Becker naevus
3. Congenital blue naevus

CONGENITAL MELANOCYTIC NAEVUS

Diagnosis

Congenital melanocytic naevi (CMN), also called giant hairy naevus

Discussion

Congenital melanocytic naevi (CMN) are benign, pigmented, melanocytic naevi present at birth. They are macular at birth. Some CMN lesions are either invisible or barely visible at birth, and then become clinically apparent in the first year of life—these are termed "tardive". These "darken" as they fully appear over a period of years. There can occasionally be a tardive element to a normal CMN, in which a subtle café-au-lait colouring adjacent to the main CMN becomes darker after birth. This can give the appearance of the CMN growing out of proportion to the child, which is not the usual clinical behaviour of CMN.

In non-scalp CMN, overlying hair is often not apparent at birth and may develop in the first year. Scalp CMN often have thick luxuriant or wiry hair at birth. Benign proliferative nodules or rhabdomyosarcoma may arise within CMN.

The lifetime risk of melanoma in all sizes of CMN is 0.1–2%. However, if the patient has more than one CMN, or a single naevus of >60 cm PAS (projected adult size) the risks of neurological and malignant complications (10–14%) are high. Identified neurological abnormalities are seizures (commonly temporal lobe epilepsy), neurodevelopmental delay, attention deficit hyperactivity disorder, hydrocephalus, and autistic spectrum disorder (Kinsler & Sebire, 2016, 75.9).

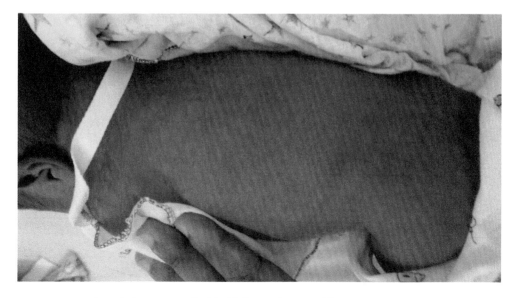

FIGURE 1.4   A newborn baby presented with this hyperpigmented lesion.

Investigations

This is a clinical diagnosis. Further investigations are planned according to predicted complications. MRI scans are recommended if the patient has seizures. The commonest site for intraparenchymal melanosis is the amygdala; therefore, the seizures are most commonly temporal lobe epilepsy.

Management

- Careful clinical, neurological history and examination after birth is important.
- Referral to a paediatric neurologist for further assessment is recommended. Any child with clinical abnormalities should have an MRI of the CNS. In the absence of abnormal clinical neurology, children with a single CMN (independent of size or site) do not require routine MRI of the CNS. Children with multiple (i.e., two or more) CMN at birth (independent of size or site) should have a routine MRI of the brain and whole spine with contrast injection, preferably within the first 6 months (Jahnke et al., 2021).
- From the cosmetic viewpoint, management is dependent on the individual:
  - Hair can be removed most easily by shaving, which may not have to be done very often to improve the appearance significantly. Hair removal creams and waxing are usually too harsh to use on CMN in children, causing irritation or skin removal.
  - Superficial removal techniques such as dermabrasion or curettage or laser therapy can be effective.
  - Serial excision of single lesions or cosmetically prominent lesions (e.g., on the face) can produce very good results although inevitably will leave a scar (Gout, 2023).
  - Some centres favour large-scale removal using balloon skin expansion techniques, and cosmetic results can also be excellent (Stefanaki et al., 2016, 132.15).

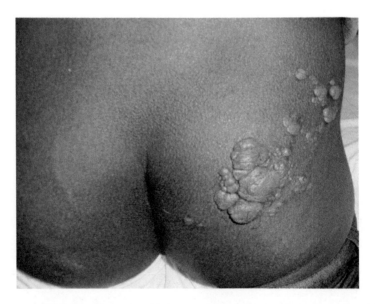

FIGURE 1.5   A 12-year-old girl wanted to get this lump removed. This had been there since birth and progressively enlarged over the years.

Based on the case description and Figure 1.5, what are your differential diagnoses?

1. Connective tissue naevus
2. Lymphangioma
3. Lipoma

CONNECTIVE TISSUE NAEVUS (COLLAGEN NAEVUS)

Diagnosis

Connective tissue naevus (collagen naevus)

Discussion

Congenital connective tissue naevi are a clinically heterogeneous group of hamartomas, named by the predominant cell type on histology, and therefore usually require biopsy for accurate diagnosis.

These lesions present at birth, although the average age for presentation of any connective tissue naevus is 2 years.

Congenital collagenomas are soft to firm, skin-coloured, brownish, or yellowish nodules or plaques. They can be single or multiple, and can be associated with extracutaneous features: plantar collagenomas are seen in both Proteus syndrome and PIK3CA overgrowth syndromes (Kinsler & Sebire, 2016, 75.17).

Investigations

Histopathology for accurate phenotypic diagnosis

Management

Debulking surgery was performed with favourable cosmetic outcome.

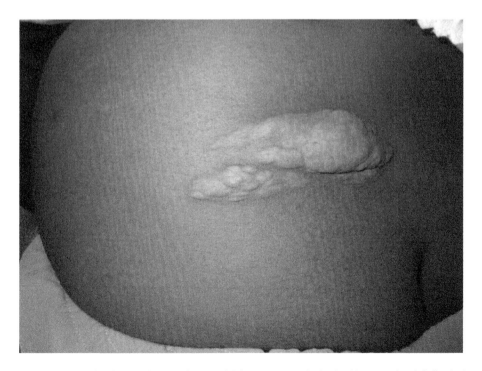

FIGURE 1.6   A 10-year-old obese girl wanted to get this lump removed. This had been on her left flank since birth.

Based on the case description and Figure 1.6, what are your differential diagnoses?

1. Connective tissue naevus
2. Plexiform neurofibroma
3. Lipoma

CONNECTIVE TISSUE NAEVUS (CONGENITAL LIPOMA)

Diagnosis

Connective tissue naevus (congenital lipoma)

Discussion

Congenital lipomas present as localized, skin-coloured, soft proliferations with indistinct edges. Histopathological examination of a full-thickness skin biopsy is often useful for accurate diagnosis of connective tissue naevi, with adjacent normal skin being helpful for comparison. When congenital lipomas lie in the lumbosacral area an underlying spinal defects should be sought using appropriate imaging techniques (Kinsler & Sebire, 2016, 75.17).

Investigations

Histopathology for accurate phenotypic diagnosis
MRI and/or ultrasonography to assess underlying spinal defects if the lesion overlying the spine

Management

Debulking surgery was performed with favourable cosmetic outcome.

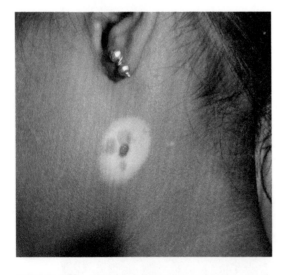

FIGURE 1.7A This skin lesion appeared over a month on a 10-year-old girl. Her mother could remember that the child has had a black naevus there before.

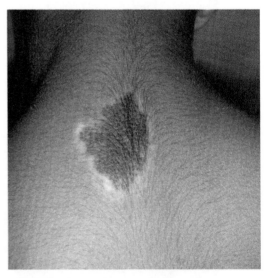

FIGURE 1.7B Depigmented halo appearing around a congenital melanocytic naevus.

Based on the case description and Figure 1.7, what are your differential diagnoses?

1. Halo naevus
2. Vitiligo

HALO NAEVUS OR SUTTON NAEVUS

Diagnosis

Halo naevus or Sutton naevus

Discussion

A halo naevus is a melanocytic naevus surrounded by a rim of depigmentation. Halo naevi can be associated with autoimmune disorders like vitiligo, Hashimoto thyroiditis, alopecia areata, and atopic eczema. Within months the naevus may gradually shrink or even disappear completely, leaving a white macule. The depigmented area usually persists for a decade or longer.

Investigations

This is a clinical diagnosis.

Management

In children and adults no treatment is required. Reassurance.

A halo naevus presenting in an older patient should raise concern, especially in the absence of vitiligo and no history of halo naevi in the past. In such cases, a thorough skin and lymph node examination is recommended to exclude melanoma elsewhere.

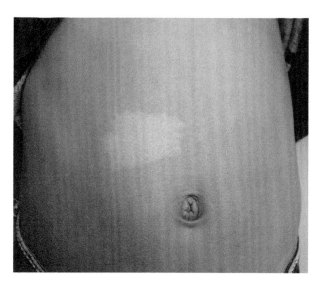

FIGURE 1.8 A 2-year-old child's mother wanted to know the sequel of this depigmented patch. This had been noticed since infancy, and has not grown out of proportion to the child's growth.

Based on the case description and Figure 1.8, what are your differential diagnoses?

1. Vitiligo
2. Hypomelanosis of Ito
3. Depigmented/hypopigmented naevus
4. Leprosy

HYPOPIGMENTED NAEVUS

Diagnosis

Congenital depigmented or hypopigmented naevus

Discussion

These congenital, asymptomatic, depigmented skin patches are not uncommon in clinically normal dark-skinned babies. These are isolated lesions, not associated with any systemic abnormalities (excluding syndromes), do not follow Blaschko's lines (excluding hypomelanosis of Ito), repigmentation is never a feature (excluding piebaldism), do not change in colour, texture, or size over the period, and are not inherited.

After extensive literature review authors could not find description of these in publications (Ranawaka, 2021a). Possible explanation is that even though these are easily visible in darker skin, since the affected individuals are clinically normal these may go unnoticed in white skin. Current textbooks show minimal skin type diversity, with only 4.5% of images showing dark skin; therefore, skin problems confined to darker skin are ignored in most of today's text books (Louie & Wilkes, 2018; Ebede & Papier, 2006).

Investigations

This is a clinical diagnosis.

Management

None, reassurance is adequate.

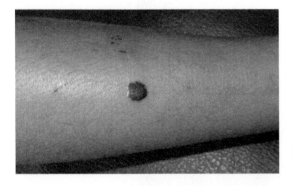

FIGURE 1.9A A 7-year-old girl has had this black lump on her leg for more than a year. Her mother had noticed a recent growth.

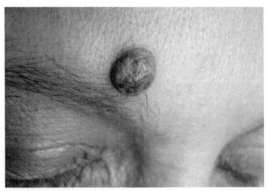

FIGURE 1.9B Intradermal (or dermal) naevus in an adult.

Based on the case description and Figure 1.9a, what are your differential diagnoses?

1. Acquired melanocytic naevus
2. Congenital melanocytic naevus
3. Melanoma (almost unseen in darker-skinned children)

MOLE

Diagnosis

Acquired melanocytic naevi (mole)

Discussion

Acquired melanocytic naevi are a benign proliferation of melanocytes that changes morphology depending on the level of skin involvement. They begin to proliferate at the dermal–epidermal junction (junctional naevus), and over time tend to migrate into the dermis while a component remains in contact with the basal layer (compound naevus). At the end stage of this process, all the naevus cells are completely detached from the overlying epidermis (intradermal naevus) (Stefanaki et al., 2016, 132.18).

Clinically, the junctional naevus presents as a uniformly pigmented dark black macule, with a diameter of 2–10 mm, and are found anywhere in the body. A compound naevus is a dark black, slightly raised, oval or round papule with symmetrical shape. Intradermal (or dermal) naevi are dark black-coloured, dome-shaped nodules that can be larger than junctional naevi. Their surface is usually smooth but can also appear papillomatous.

Melanoma or naevi transforming into melanoma are almost unseen in dark skin children.

Management

No treatment is required. Surgical removal is performed only for aesthetic purposes.

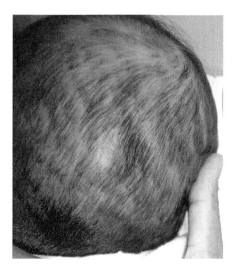

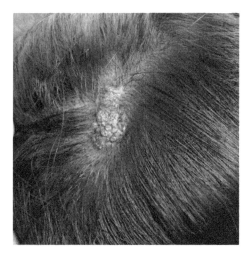

FIGURE 1.10A This newborn baby had an erythematous patch on the scalp since birth. On examination, verrucous raised waxy surface noticed.

FIGURE 1.10B A 12-year-old girl came with this progressively growing verrucous plaque on the scalp. Her mother admits that there was a palpable skin lesion at the site since birth.

Based on the case description and Figure 1.10a, what are your differential diagnoses?

1. Naevus sebaceous
2. Infantile haemangioma

Diagnosis

Diagnosis was not confirmed in this baby.

Discussion

Even though the histopathology may confirm the diagnosis, skin biopsy is avoided in infancy and in small children. Therefore, the parents were educated, and the baby was kept under observation for the progression of the lesion.

Management

Keep under observation for the progression of the lesion.
    Based on the case description and Figure 1.10b, what are your differential diagnoses?

1. Naevus sebaceous
2. Verrucous epidermal naevus
3. Viral wart

NAEVUS SEBACEOUS

Diagnosis

Naevus sebaceous

Discussion

Sebaceous naevi are congenital epidermal naevi (CEN) of sebaceous gland origin. They have a greasy feel and appearance, are often yellowish or brown at birth, but can sometimes be deeply pigmented. They usually present in childhood as a hairless patch on the scalp (Figure 1.10a), often in a linear configuration. At puberty, the lesion becomes more prominent with particular increase in the size of the sebaceous glands. For single isolated sebaceous naevus, the risk of malignant transformation is approximately 1%; syringocystadenoma papilliferum is the commonest, whereas basal cell carcinoma occurs in less than 1% and squamous cell carcinoma is rare (Lee et al., 2022).

Investigations

Biopsy and histopathology for confirmation

Management

Ablative laser therapy to reduce the thickness and/or hyperkeratosis of the lesion, and smaller verrucous lesions have been treated successfully with cryotherapy.

Complete excision gives better cosmetic results.

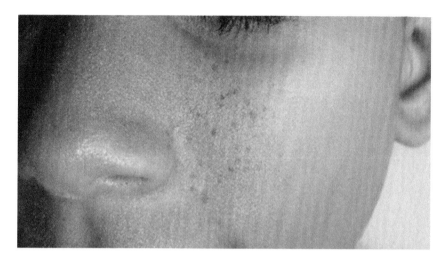

FIGURE 1.11   A 9-year-old boy's mother is worried that darkly pigmented patches are developing on one area of the face. They have noted a slight colour difference on that area before, but that was not noticeable in his dark brown skin.

Based on the case description and Figure 1.11, what are your differential diagnoses?

1. Naevus spillus
2. Segmental lentiginosis
3. Café-au-lait spot

NAEVUS SPILLUS

Diagnosis

Naevus spillus or speckled lentiginous naevus

Discussion

Naevus spillus or speckled lentiginous naevus (SLN) is a congenital melanocytic naevus. It presents as a lentiginous macule early in life—at birth or during early childhood—and later develops multiple darkly pigmented macules or papules in a speckled distribution. This macular stage goes unnoticed in dark skin, and only when they develop blackish spots do patients seek medical advice. Mostly, SLN is benign and uncomplicated.

Occasionally, SLN can be a part of complex disorders such as speckled lentiginous naevus syndrome (SLN syndrome), phakomatosis pigmentovascularis (PPV) or phakomatosis pigmentokeratotica (PPK). SLN syndrome is characterized by a papular SLN associated with ipsilateral neuromuscular, peripheral nerve, and/or central nervous system defects. PPV is characterized by the coexistence of a macular SLN with a pale pink telangiectatic naevus. PPK is characterized by the presence of a sebaceous naevus and a papular SLN, with or without skeletal and neurological disturbances (Stefanaki et al., 2016, 132.15).

A few cases of melanoma arising within SLN have been reported, but the risk is very low.

Investigations

This is a clinical diagnosis.

Management

The patient is instructed to monitor the naevus for suspicious lesions.

Excision, ablative and non-ablative lasers, and dermabrasion are used for cosmetic reasons.

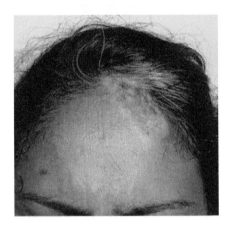

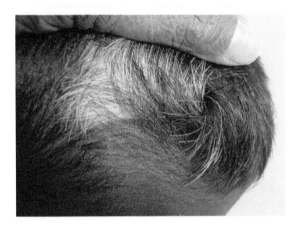

FIGURE 1.12A This girl wanted to know availabilities of newer therapies for this depigmented patch which she has had since birth. She admits that her paternal relatives have similar skin patches.

FIGURE 1.12B This 8-year-old boy's complaint was a recently appeared flock of white hair on the scalp. On examination, a vitiligo patch on the underlying scalp was detected. This is a case of vitiligo with poliosis or leukotrichia.

Based on the case description and Figure 1.12a, what are your differential diagnoses?

1. Piebaldism
2. Vitiligo with leukotrichia (white hair)
3. Poliosis (depigmented hair)
4. Segmental vitiligo

PIEBALDISM

Diagnosis

Piebaldism

Discussion

Piebaldism is a rare autosomal dominant trait characterized by well-demarcated irregular hypopigmented macules The most typical and common clinical feature of piebaldism is a white forelock, often associated with a V-shaped area of leukoderma on the mid-forehead. Often, white patches occur on the upper chest, abdomen, and limbs, bilaterally but not necessarily symmetrically. In addition, small spots of hyperpigmentation arise subsequently within the hypopigmented lesions or at the edge of the lesion.

If the interpupillary distance is increased or the patient is deaf, the diagnosis of Waardenburg syndrome must be considered. Waardenburg syndrome is an autosomal dominant genetic disorder characterized by piebaldism and sensorineural deafness.

Piebaldism can be distinguished from **vitiligo** because of the neonatal presence of white patches. Overall, piebaldism lesions remain stable in adults.

Poliosis is defined as the presence of a localized patch of white hair resulting from the absence or deficiency of melanin in a group of neighbouring follicles. Pigment absence can be congenital or acquired. Acquired forms of poliosis are due to vitiligo or to regrowth of non-pigmented hair following alopecia areata.

Investigations

This is a clinical diagnosis. Piebaldism and vitiligo are clinically indistinguishable especially when there is a single vitiligo patch. Piebaldism is inherited autosomal dominant while vitiligo is acquired.

Management

The evolution of piebaldism is benign.

Sun protection is recommended to protect the amelanotic areas from burning.

Epidermal cell or skin grafting have been successfully tried (Taieb et al., 2016, 70.3).

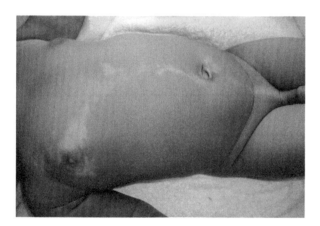

FIGURE 1.13   A 6-month-old baby had this asymptomatic hypopigmented patch since birth, which was more conspicuous since 2 months of age. The child was clinically and developmentally normal.

Based on the case description and Figure 1.13, what are your differential diagnoses?

1. Segmental vitiligo
2. Pigmentary mosaicism
3. Piebaldism
4. Hypomelanosis of Ito

PIGMENTARY MOSAICISM

Diagnosis

Pigmentary mosaicism

Discussion

At birth most brown babies are pinkish and fairer. Therefore, some inherited or congenital hypopigmented lesions may go unnoticed at birth. These become apparent when their skin regains darker colour in a few weeks after birth.

Pigmentary mosaicism is a genetically determined variation of skin pigmentation. It often presents as streaks and whorls of hypo- or hyperpigmentation following Blaschko's lines with midline demarcation. Pigmentary mosaicism may also manifest as patches, flag-like, leaf-like, or chequerboard shapes, or as patchy variation without midline demarcation. It may be found in association with neurological and musculoskeletal deformities. Infants with pigmentary mosaicism should be assessed for development, the internal organs, and skeletal and ophthalmological abnormalities.

One special type of chromosomal mosaicism is the hypomelanosis of Ito (Stefanaki et al., 2016, 132.14). **Hypomelanosis of Ito** is a rare neuroectodermal disorder often associated with mental retardation and epilepsy. Unilateral or bilateral cutaneous macular hypopigmented whorls, streaks, and patches, corresponding to the lines of Blaschko. Extracutaneous findings include neurological, ophthalmological, and skeletal defects. (Taieb et al., 2016, 70.10)

Investigations

This is a clinical diagnosis. Investigations are performed if any neurological, ophthalmological, or skeletal defects are detected.

Management

None; reassure parents.

HAEMANGIOMAS

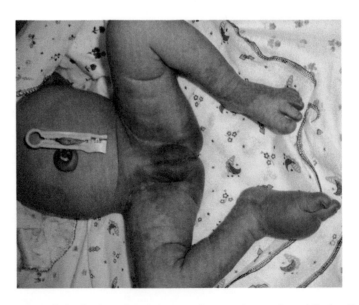

FIGURE 1.14 A new-born baby had erythematous patches on the trunk and limbs. Careful examination revealed asymmetrical growth of limbs: right lower limb was swollen and was longer than the left.

Based on the case description and Figure 1.14, what are your differential diagnoses?

1. Capillary malformation–arteriovenous malformation (CM-AVM)
2. Parkes Weber syndrome

A-V MALFORMATION

Diagnosis

Capillary malformation–arteriovenous malformation (CM-AVM)

Discussion

Capillary malformation–arteriovenous malformation (CM-AVM) is an autosomal dominant disorder characterized by multifocal CMs and an increased risk for fast-flow vascular malformations, either arteriovenous malformation (AVM) or, arteriovenous fistula (AVF). All affected individuals have multiple, multifocal cutaneous capillary malformations. The AVMs and AVFs may be located within the central nervous system (intracranial or intraspinal) or out sides (limbs, face, and neck). They may have symptoms of cardiac failure, hydrocephaly, epilepsy, developmental delay, para- or tetraplegia, and neurogenic bladder.

Parkes Weber syndrome is capillary blush on an upper or lower extremity, bony and soft tissue hypertrophy, and multiple arteriolar-venular microfistulae. The major problem associated with Parkes Weber syndrome is leg length discrepancy causing scoliosis.

Investigations

This is a clinical diagnosis. The AVMs/AVFs are followed by Doppler ultrasound and/or MRI and arteriography. Leg length discrepancy in patients with Parkes Weber syndrome is followed radiographically. Genetic consultation is needed to assess family history, and genetic testing can confirm the clinical diagnosis.

Management

Patients with AVM should be followed by a multidisciplinary team specializing in vascular anomalies. The risks and benefits to treat or not are based on symptoms, patient age, lesion size and location, angioarchitecture and expected evolution. The limb length discrepancy is monitored until the end of puberty.

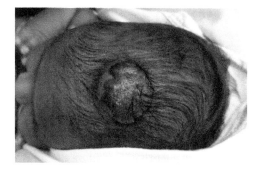

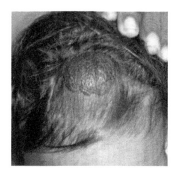

FIGURE 1.15A A 3-week-old baby was brought with this lesion. Ultrasonography of the scalp was performed to assess the intracranial extension. Note, in very dark skin the haemangioma may appear dark red to blackish.

FIGURE 1.15B The same baby girl at 10 months of age. She was treated with oral propranolol considering the possibility of invisible intracranial extension.

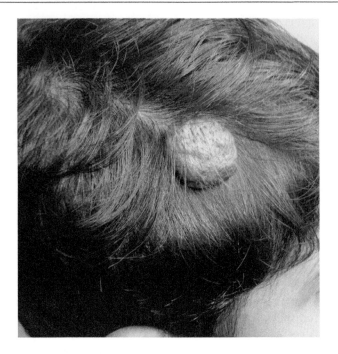

FIGURE 1.15C   A non-involuting haemangioma on the scalp in a 3-year-old girl.

Based on the case description and Figure 1.15a, what are your differential diagnoses?

1. Infantile haemangioma
2. Arterio-venous malformation

INFANTILE HAEMANGIOMA

Diagnosis

Infantile haemangioma

Discussion

Infantile haemangiomas are the most common benign vascular tumours in infancy. The natural history is proliferation in the first few months of life, and involution over the next 3–7 years. Most resolve spontaneously without sequelae. Infantile haemangiomas of the head and neck and of the lumbosacral region may be associated with structural anomalies. Multifocal infantile haemangiomas are usually asymptomatic but may be associated with extensive visceral involvement. The main complications are ulceration, disfigurement, and functional impairment that depend on the location and the size of the lesion (Ranawaka, 2021b).

Investigations

This is a clinical diagnosis.

The distinction between infantile haemangiomas and vascular malformations is often straightforward on the basis of history and examination, but occasionally investigations such as ultrasound, histopathology, and immunohistochemistry are required. Relevant investigations are performed to assess functional impairments (Macca et al., 2022).

Management (Léauté-Labrèze et al., 2008)

- For small lesions no treatment is required.
- Infantile haemangiomas causing or likely to cause impairment of function or permanent disfigurement are treated.
- Non-selective β-blockade with topical timolol or systemic propranolol has become the treatment of choice for proliferative haemangiomas, especially complicated lesions on the face, near the eye, or those with the potential of causing respiratory embarrassment. Topical propranolol 1% twice daily is prescribed for superficial infantile haemangiomas. The use of one drop of timolol maleate 0.5% gel forming solution (GFS) up to three times a day to non-ulcerated, non-mucosal lesions appears to be safe. Although β-blockers may be helpful for the treatment of ulcerated infantile haemangioma, worsening of ulceration can occur, perhaps reflecting reduced blood flow (Chang et al., 2022; Higgins & Glover, 2016).
- Pulsed dye laser (PDL) or Nd:YAG lasers can be helpful for the treatment in ulcerated, involuting haemangiomas, and may be used for telangiectases and erythema post-involution, though ulceration is itself a rare complication of treatment.
- Surgery may very occasionally be required for infantile haemangioma in the proliferative phase if functional impairment or ulceration cannot be managed medically.
- Embolization may have a role for life-threatening haemangiomas or those leading to congestive cardiac failure that have not responded to medical therapy (Novoa et al., 2018).

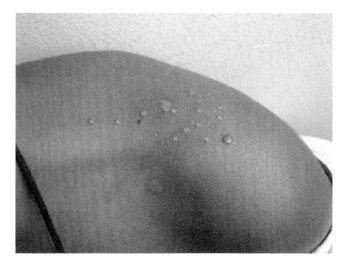

FIGURE 1.16   A 7-year-old girl came with this small vesicular rash on her left shoulder where new vesicles were appearing over a year.

Based on the case description and Figure 1.16, what are your differential diagnoses?

1. Molluscum contagiosum
2. Lymphangioma circumscriptum

LYMPHANGIOMA

Diagnosis

Lymphangioma circumscriptum

Discussion

Lymphangioma or lymphatic malformations are the result of abnormal development of lymphatics during embryogenesis and fetal life. These may be single-vessel forms or a combination (capillary, arterial, lymphatic, and venous). Localized congenital lymphatic malformations can be macrocystic (deep) or microcystic (superficial) lesions, or a combination. The macrocystic swellings containing clear lymph are called cystic hygromas. Most occur in the neck and may extend into the upper mediastinum, also in the groin.

Lymphangioma circumscriptum is a lymphatic malformation that is superficial and localized to an area of skin, subcutaneous tissue, and sometimes muscle. Lymphangioma circumscriptum manifest as fluid-filled vesicles ("lymph blisters"), which bulge on the skin surface. They may be translucent, appearing at birth or during infancy either as a localized subcutaneous swelling or as "frogspawn" (groups of watery or haemorrhagic vesicles or lymph blisters) on the skin. The most common complications are recurrent oozing (lymphorrhoea) and cellulitis.

Investigations

This is a clinical diagnosis. Histopathology is performed for confirmation. It shows marked expanded channels in the dermis, which can extend into the subcutaneous and other deeper tissues. The channels are lined with flattened cells, which express CD31 and D2-40 (Mortimer & Gordon, 2016, 105.34).

Management

- Surface vesicles that weep or bleed should be destroyed by diathermy or laser.
- Infection should be treated promptly with antibiotics, as in lymphoedema.
- If recurrent attacks of infection occur, then prophylactic antibiotics should be considered.
- Sclerotherapy is the mainstay of treatment of macrocystic lymphatic malformations, but the response using traditional sclerosants is much less beneficial in microcystic lesions.
- Debulking procedures may be necessary for very large malformations causing complications such as the obstruction of vital organs and their functions.
- Sildenafil can reduce lymphatic malformation, volume, and symptoms in some children.

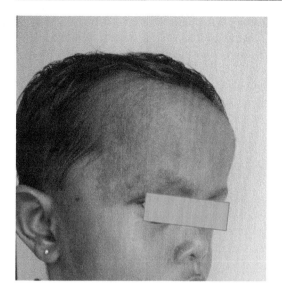

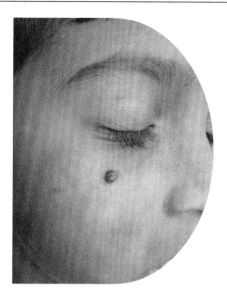

FIGURE 1.17A A 4-year-old girl came with this erythematous patch on the forehead. The mother had noticed that this becomes more reddish when she cries, eats hot spices, and has sun exposure. Direct inquiry revealed that there had been a difference in skin colour in this area since birth.

FIGURE 1.17B Pyogenic granuloma appeared on top of port wine stain in a 5-year-old boy. Note erythema is very faint and easily missed in darker skin.

Based on the case description and Figure 1.17, what are your differential diagnoses?

1. Port wine stain
2. Sturge–Weber syndrome (SWS)

PORT WINE STAIN

Diagnosis

Port wine stain (PWS, congenital superficial capillary malformations)

Discussion

PWS is a capillary malformation (CM), and is the most common vascular malformation. The incidence is around 1:1000 with equal sex distribution. It is characterized by pink, red, or purple flat lesions of variable size and with geographic borders. It is usually located on the head and neck, but can also be seen on the trunk or limbs. A CM grows proportionately with the child and persists throughout life. PWSs thicken diffusely over time with approximately two thirds of patients developing hypertrophic or nodular lesions by age 50 years (Dompmartin et al., 2016, 73.1). Most lesions are uncomplicated. However, associated signs and symptoms, large size, and multifocality evoke a possible "syndromic" form. For example, on the upper face, the larger the lesion, the higher the risk for Sturge–Weber syndrome.

Sturge–Weber syndrome (SWS) describes PWS involving skin in the distribution of the ophthalmic branch of the trigeminal nerve (V1), together with ipsilateral ocular choroid and leptomeninges involvement. Patients with a periorbital PWS should also be tested for glaucoma.

Investigations

This is a clinical diagnosis. Most CMs do not require any investigation. However, if SWS is suspected, brain magnetic resonance imaging (MRI), an ophthalmological evaluation of the fundus of the eye, and regular assessment of intraocular pressure are necessary (Dompmartin et al., 2010).

Management

- Pulsed dye laser (PDL) is the intervention of choice for uncomplicated lesions and 6–8 treatments spaced at 4–6-week intervals will achieve "good results" in as many as 60%. Laser treatment consists of several consecutive sessions. Due to pain, general anaesthesia is often used for children.
- Longer wavelength, variable pulse width lasers such as the alexandrite 810 nm diode and 1064 nm Nd:YAG lasers and IPL systems can be used to treat resistant or recurrent PWSs.
- Adult patients in whom progressive vascular ectasia has resulted in very exophytic lesions are best treated with a CO_2 laser (Madan & Barlow, 2016, 23.6).
- Management of epilepsy and glaucoma is an emergency.

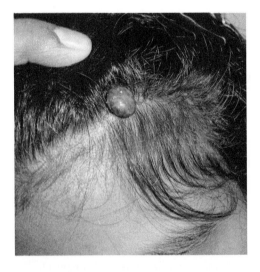

FIGURE 1.18A A 9-year-old girl came with this erythematous lump which had appeared within one month.

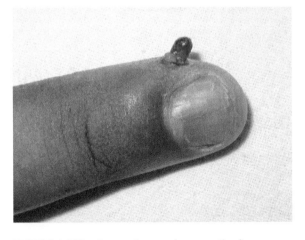

FIGURE 1.18B Pyogenic granuloma on the finger.

Based on the case description and Figure 1.18a, what are your differential diagnoses?

1. Pyogenic granuloma
2. Amelanotic melanoma
3. Malignant deposits

PYOGENIC GRANULOMA

Diagnosis

Pyogenic granuloma

Discussion

Pyogenic granuloma is a common acquired benign vascular tumour. It is bright red to brownish-red or blue-black in colour. It is partially compressible, but cannot be completely blanched, does not show pulsation, and may bleed very easily. Spontaneous disappearance is rare. This can clinically mimic keratoacanthoma and other epithelial neoplasms, inflamed seborrhoeic keratoses, melanocytic naevi, melanoma and Spitz naevi, viral warts, molluscum contagiosum, angioma, glomus tumour, eccrine poroma, Kaposi sarcoma, and metastatic carcinoma.

Pyogenic granulomatous-like lesions may occur in severe acne and acne fulminans, result from treatment with isotretinoin, or occur in association with hidradenitis suppurativa. These lesions may respond to clobetasol propionate cream applied topically twice daily and carefully to the lesions over a 2–3-week period (Layton et al., 2016, 90.36)

Investigations

Complete excision and histopathology are recommended to exclude malignant clinical mimics.

Management

- Simple excision is the treatment of choice, because lesions do not regress spontaneously. Local recurrence may be seen after incomplete excision.
- The pedunculated lesions are easy to treat by curettage with cauterization or diathermy coagulation of the base.
- Other treatment modalities that have been used are topical imiquimod 5% cream both in children and adults with complete resolution, Nd:YAG laser, cryosurgery, intralesional steroids, flash lamp pulsed dye laser, sclerotherapy with sodium tetra decyl sulphate, and even injection of absolute ethanol.

REFERENCES

Al-Bakaa MK, Al-Dhalimi MA, Dube P, Khalaf FK (2022). Evaluating the roles of different types of laser therapy in becker's nevus treatment. *Journal of Clinical Medicine* 21;11(14):4230. doi: 10.3390/jcm11144230.

Chang SJ, Chang HF, Qiu Y, et al. (2022). Does oral propranolol improve the final outcome of all involuted infantile hemangiomas? A matched retrospective comparative study. *Annals of Plastic Surgery* 1;89(2):214–7.

Dompmartin A, Revencu N, Boon LM, et al. (2016). Disorders affecting cutaneous vasculature. In Christopher G, Jonathan B, Tanya B, Robert C, Daniel C, eds. *Rook's Textbook of Dermatology*, 9th edn. Hoboken: Wiley-Blackwell, 73.2p.

Dompmartin A, Vikkula M, Boon LM (2010). Venous malformation: Update on aetiopathogenesis, diagnosis and management. *Phlebology* 25(5):224–35. doi: 10.1258/phleb.2009.009041.

Ebede T, Papier A (2006). Disparities in dermatology educational resources. *The Journal of the American Academy of Dermatology*;55(4):687–90. doi: 10.1016/j.jaad.2005.10.068.

Gout HA, Fledderus AC, Lokhorst MM, et al. (2023). Safety and effectiveness of surgical excision of medium, large, and giant congenital melanocytic nevi: A systematic review and meta-analysis. *Journal of Plastic, Reconstructive and Aesthetic Surgery*;77:430–55. doi: 10.1016/j.bjps.2022.10.048.

Gupta D, Thappa DM (2013). Mongolian spots–A prospective study. *Pediatric Dermatology*;30(6):683–8. doi: 10.1111/pde.12191.

Higgins EM, Glover MT (2016). Dermatoses and haemangiomas of infancy. In Christopher G, Jonathan B, Tanya B, Robert C, Daniel C, eds. *Rook's Textbook of Dermatology*, 9th edn. Hoboken: Wiley-Blackwell, 117.12p.

Jahnke MN, O'Haver J, Gupta D, et al. (2021). Care of congenital melanocytic nevi in newborns and infants: Review and management recommendations. *Pediatrics* 1;148(6):e2021051536.

Kinsler VA, Sebire NJ (2016). Congenital naevi and other developmental abnormalities affecting the skin. In Christopher G, Jonathan B, Tanya B, Robert C, Daniel C, eds. R*ook's Textbook of Dermatology*, 9th edn. Hoboken: Wiley-Blackwell, 75.3p, 75.14p.

Layton AM, Eady EA, Zouboulis CC (2016). Acne. In Christopher G, Jonathan B, Tanya B, Robert C, Daniel C, eds. *Rook's Textbook of Dermatology*, 9th edn. Hoboken: Wiley-Blackwell, 90.36p.

Léauté-Labrèze C, et al. (2008). Propranolol for severe hemangiomas of infancy. *The New England Journal of Medicine* 12;358(24):2649–51.

Lee YJ, Han HJ, Kim DY, et al. (2022). Malignant transformation of nevus sebaceous to basal-cell carcinoma: Case series, literature review, and management algorithm. Medicine (Baltimore) 5;101(31):e29988. doi: 10.1097/MD.0000000000029988.

Louie P, Wilkes R (2018). Representations of race and skin tone in medical textbook imagery. *Social Science & Medicine*;202:38–42. doi: 10.1016/j.socscimed.2018.02.023.

Macca L, Altavilla D, Di Bartolomeo L, et al. (2022). Update on treatment of infantile hemangiomas: What's new in the last five years? *Front Pharmacol* 26;13:879602.

Madan V, Barlow RJ (2016). Principles of cutaneous laser therapy. In Christopher G, Jonathan B, Tanya B, Robert C, Daniel C, eds. *Rook's Textbook of Dermatology*, 9th edn. Hoboken: Wiley-Blackwell, 23.6p.

Mortimer PS, Gordon K (2016). Disorders of the lymphatic vessels. In Christopher G, Jonathan B, Tanya B, Robert C, Daniel C, eds. *Rook's Textbook of Dermatology*, 9th edn. Hoboken: Wiley-Blackwell, 105.34p.

Novoa M, et al. (2018). Interventions for infantile haemangiomas of the skin. *Cochrane Database Systematic Reviews* 18;4(4):CD006545. doi: 10.1002/14651858.CD006545.pub3.

Paasch U, Zidane M, Baron JM, et al. (2022). S2k guideline: Laser therapy of the skin. *Journal Der Deutschen Dermatologischen Gesellschaft*;20(9):1248–67. doi: 10.1111/ddg.14879.

Ranawaka RR (2021a). Congenital naevi and melanocytic naevi. In Ranawaka RR, Kannangara AP, Karawita A, eds. *Atlas of Dermatoses in Pigmented Skin*. Singapore: Springer, pp. 49–64. doi: 10.1007/978-981-15-5483-4_2

Ranawaka RR (2021b). Vascular tumours and malformations. In Ranawaka RR, Kannangara AP, Karawita A, eds. *Atlas of Dermatoses in Pigmented Skin*. Singapore: Springer, pp. 65–80. doi: 10.1007/978-981-15-5483-4_3

Stefanaki I, Antoniou C, Stratigos A (2016). Benign melanocytic proliferations and melanocytic naevi. In Christopher G, Jonathan B, Tanya B, Robert C, Daniel C, eds. *Rook's Textbook of Dermatology*, 9th edn. Hoboken: Wiley-Blackwell, 132.18p.

Taieb A, Morice-Picard F, Ezzedine K (2016). Genetic disorders of pigmentation. In Christopher G, Jonathan B, Tanya B, Robert C, Daniel C, eds. *Rook's Textbook of Dermatology*, 9th edn. Hoboken: Wiley-Blackwell, 70.10p.

Infections in Children with FST 5

2

Ajith P. Kannangara and Ranthilaka R. Gammanpila

INTRODUCTION

This chapter discusses 23 common skin infections we encounter in children with brown skin (Fitzpatrick skin type V/FST 5) using 51 clinical photographs. These are discussed based on a clinical photograph and easy-to-read question-and-answer format.

Erythema is inconspicuous and post-inflammatory hypopigmentation and hyperpigmentation are marked in coloured-skinned children. For example, the first sign of erythema or macular, orange-red, scarlatiniform eruption can be inconspicuous and can be easily missed in darker-skinned babies with SSSS leading to delayed diagnosis, more complications and high mortality in an inexperienced setting; erythrasma is never erythematous in darker-skinned babies.

BACTERIAL

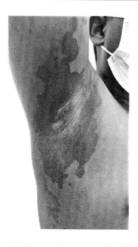

FIGURE 2.1 A 15-year-old boy came with hyperpigmented discolouration of axillary area for one year. (Photographed by Ajith P. Kannangara.)

DOI: 10.1201/9781003321507-2

Based on the clinical history and Figure 2.1, what is your differential diagnosis?

1. Erythrasma
2. Acanthosis nigricans
3. Hyperpigmented pityriasis versicolor
4. Confluent and reticulated papillomatosis

ERYTHRASMA

Diagnosis

Erythrasma.

Discussion

Erythrasma is a superficial, localized, non-pyogenic skin infection caused by *Corynebacterium minutissimum*. The organism produces coproporphyrin III as a metabolic product which gives the reddish fluorescence. It is common in obese adults and diabetic patients. Axillae, groins, sub-mammary regions, and toe-web spaces are the common sites of involvement. The lesion occurs as reddish brown (in fairer skin) or dark brown (in darker skin), scaly asymptomatic, or mildly pruritic patch of long duration (Forouzan & Cohen, 2020).

Investigation

Wood's lamp examination of the unwashed involved sites reveals "coral red fluorescence", but Wood's lamp is not necessary to diagnose erythrasma in brown skin.

Management

Topical clotrimazole/miconazole or Fucidin is the initial treatment. If response is inadequate or there are extensive lesions, oral erythromycin can be administered.

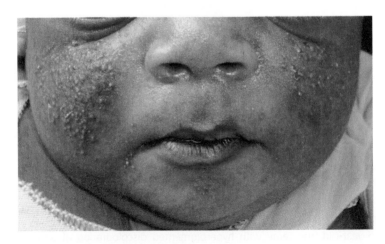

FIGURE 2.2A A 2-week-old infant was brought with vesicular, pustular eruption on both cheeks. The child was afebrile and was clinically well. (Photographed by Dr. Ranthilaka R. Gammanpila.)

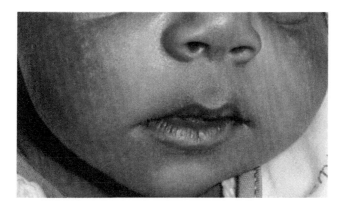

FIGURE 2.2B   After one week of topical Fucidin cream the lesions disappeared completely leaving post-inflammatory hypopigmentation that resolved spontaneously. (Photographed by Dr. Ranthilaka R. Gammanpila.)

Based on the clinical history and Figure 2.2a, what is your differential diagnosis?

1. Folliculitis
2. Infantile acne
3. Milia

FOLLICULITIS

Diagnosis

Folliculitis in infants

Discussion

Folliculitis is inflammation of the hair follicles; it may be caused by bacteria or fungi. These are quite common in hot humid climate in tropics. *Staphylococcus aureus* or *Streptococcus pyogenes* or a combination of both are the most common bacterial cause of these infections. They are pus-filled vesicles of 1 mm diameter. These can appear at any site but have a predilection to flexures and cheeks. If untreated this may lead to SSSS in infants.

Investigations

This is a clinical diagnosis.

Management

Treatment depends on the child's symptoms, age, and general health. It will also depend on how severe the condition is. This baby was treated with topical Fucidin cream twice daily for one week, and reviewed (Figure 2.2b).

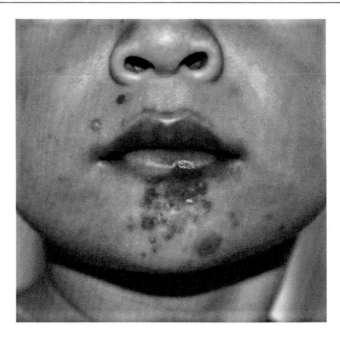

FIGURE 2.3A A 6-year-old boy presented with vesicular bullous, ulcerated lesions over the face for 3 days with mild fever. (Photographed by Dr. Ajith P. Kannangara.)

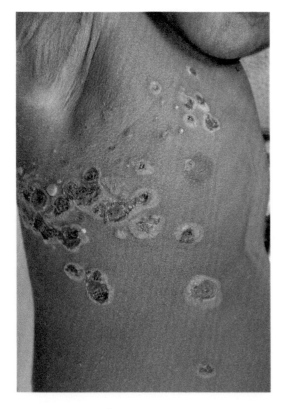

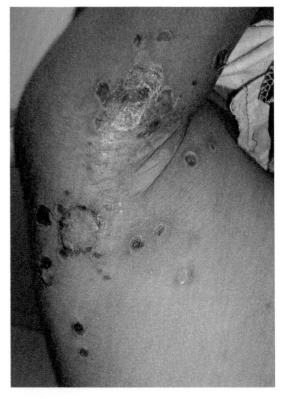

FIGURE 2.3B Bullous impetigo in an 18-month-old child. (Photographed by Dr. Ranthilaka R. Gammanpila.)

FIGURE 2.3C Non-bullous impetigo. (Photographed by Dr. Ranthilaka R. Gammanpila.)

Based on the clinical history and Figure 2.3a, what is your differential diagnosis?

1. Impetigo
2. Superficial folliculitis following insect bites
3. Herpes simplex infection
4. Miliaria crystallina

IMPETIGO

Diagnosis

Impetigo

Discussion

Impetigo is a highly contagious superficial bacterial infection, caused by *Staphylococcus aureus* or *Streptococcus pyogenes* or a combination of both. Children under 6 years are the most commonly affected. There are two types of impetigo:

A. Bullous impetigo which is caused by *Staphylococcus aureus* and mainly occurs on the face, flexures, and diaper area. The lesions are thin-walled, flaccid bullae which rupture easily to form shallow erosions. Subsequently, the erosions are covered with "varnish-like crusts".

B. Non-bullous impetigo is caused by group A *beta haemolytic streptococci*. It starts as pustules on the face and the in perioral and perinasal location above the upper lip. The lesions are erythematous and tender. "Honey-coloured crust" is seen on surface.

Investigations

Mainly clinical, and sometimes swab culture from affected site may be helpful.

Management

Prognosis of both types of impetigo is good with adequate treatment. Untreated bullous impetigo may result in generalized infection termed as staphylococcal scalded skin syndrome. Warm compress, drainage of pus, and removal of crusts are necessary for relief of symptoms. Localized impetigo can be treated with topical mupirocin ointment. Widespread skin lesions, lymphadenopathy, and fever are the indications of systemic therapy. Amoxicillin, cloxacillin, amoxicillin and clavulanic acid, cephalexin, and erythromycin are the systemic treatment options.

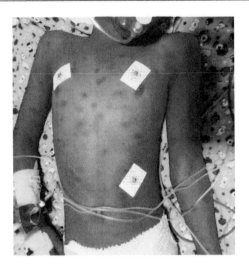

FIGURE 2.4   A 7-year-old boy presented with 3-day history of fever with generalized malaise and bit of confusion state. He has generalized petechial rash with stellate borders. (Photographed by Dr. Ajith P. Kannangara.)

Based on the clinical history and Figure 2.4, what is your differential diagnosis?

1. Meningococcal meningitis
2. Erythema multiforme
3. Other bacterial meningitis
4. Rickettsial spotted fever

MENINGOCOCCAL MENINGITIS

Diagnosis

Meningococcal meningitis

Discussion

Neisseria meningitidis is Gram-negative intracellular diplococci primarily causing meningitis. Children are more liable to be affected, and more than 50% of cases occur during infancy. Sporadic cases may occur in adults. Transmission of the organism is usually through the respiratory route. Clinical features consist of an acute-onset febrile illness causing septicaemia, meningitis, arthritis, shock, and disseminated intravascular coagulation (DIC). More than 75% of these children develop a transient erythematous rash during a febrile episode, mostly over lower extremities, palms and soles, nose, and pinna. This erythematous rash may be inconspicuous in darker-skinned patients which may cause delay in diagnosis and fatality in inexperienced hands. The lesions turn petechial, with stellate margins and vesicular or pustular centres. In severe cases, necrotic bullae and even eschar formation may occur. Purpura fulminans may develop in some cases. The organism can be isolated and cultured from the initial petechial skin lesions (Shrestha et al., 2023).

Management

Prognosis is poor, especially in the occurrence of septic shock and DIC. Acute adrenal haemorrhage (Waterhouse–Friedrichsen syndrome) is a life-threatening complication of meningococcaemia. Intravenous benzylpenicillin is the antibiotic of choice. Alternatively, ceftriaxone or cefotaxime can be used. Hemodynamic support for shock and DIC is mandatory.

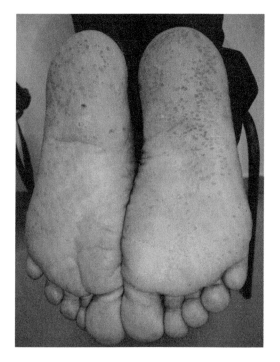

FIGURE 2.5 A 12-year-old boy complained of foul-smelling soles, especially when he removes socks after schooling. Direct inquiry revealed that he was suffering from hyperhidrosis on palms and soles. (Photographed by Dr. Ranthilaka R. Gammanpila.)

Based on the clinical history and Figure 2.5 what is your differential diagnosis?

1. Pitted keratolysis
2. Tinea pedis

PITTED KERATOLYSIS

Diagnosis

Pitted keratolysis

Discussion

This is a superficial infection of the skin apparently caused by a species of *Corynebacteria*, *Dermatophilus congolensis*, *Kytococcus sedentarius*, *Actinomyces*, or *Streptomyces*. They proliferate and produce protease enzymes that cause destruction of the stratum corneum to create pits/craters. The odour is associated with the sulfur compounds (thiols, sulphides, and thioesters) which are produced by the bacteria (Pattanaprichakul et al., 2021).

There are numerous superficial erosions of the horny layer of the soles and the undersurfaces of the toes, predominantly on pressure-bearing areas. Soaking the feet in water for 15 min causes swelling of the horny layer and accentuates the lesions. Patients often present with maceration, stickiness, and a foul odour; severe cases may be associated with pruritus and pain on walking.

Hyperhidrosis or occupations in which feet are constantly wet are at high risk: athletes, miners, farmers, sailors and fishermen, military workers, boatmen, fishmongers, swimming instructors, housewives, etc. Hyperhidrosis, obsessive compulsive disorder of washing hands and/or feet 20–30 times a day, keratoderma, and poor foot hygiene should be considered in children.

Investigations

This is a clinical diagnosis.

Management

- Topical antibiotics are the first line therapy in mild cases applied twice daily, usually for 2–4 weeks: clindamycin, erythromycin, mupirocin, or fusidic acid. Imidazoles such as clotrimazole are reputed to be effective.
- Oral antibiotics are prescribed for refractory or extensive disease: oral clindamycin or erythromycin for at least 10 days. Duration is dependent on severity and response to treatment. With treatment this often resolves in 2–4 weeks.
- Predisposing factors should be identified and dealt with: treatment of hyperhidrosis using potassium permanganate soaks, aluminum chloride, and iontophoresis. Botulinum toxin which reduces hyperhidrosis has been helpful (Ongsri et al., 2021).

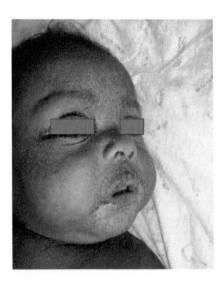

FIGURE 2.6A A 2-month-old baby was brought in complaining of fever for 2 days, generalized scaling, irritability, and poor feeding for last 24 hours. On examination, his skin was very tender to touch, generalized scaling prominently in flexures, and periorificial. (Photographed by Dr. Ranthilaka R. Gammanpila.)

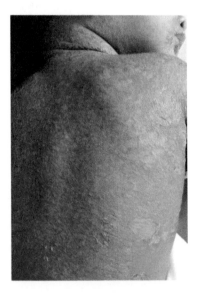

FIGURE 2.6B A 2-year-old child with SSSS. Note generalized exfoliation with positive Nikolsky's sign (the top layers of the skin slip away from the lower layers when rubbed). Nikolsky's sign is pathognomonic for pemphigus, toxic epidermal necrolysis, and staphylococcal scalded skin syndrome (SSSS). (Photographed by Dr. Ranthilaka R. Gammanpila.)

Based on the clinical history and Figure 2.6a, what is your differential diagnosis?

1. Staphylococcal scalded skin syndrome (SSSS)
2. Toxic epidermal necrolysis (TEN)

STAPHYLOCOCCAL SCALDED SKIN SYNDROME (SSSS)

Diagnosis

Staphylococcal scalded skin syndrome (SSSS)

Discussion

SSSS is caused by epidermolytic toxin A and/or B of certain strains of *Staphylococcus Aureus*, most commonly of phage group II, particularly strains 71 and 55. These toxins reach the skin via the circulation from a distant focus of infection, usually in the umbilicus, breast, conjunctiva, or the site of circumcision. Neonates are more prone, and is believed to reflect less efficient metabolism and excretion of the toxin (Gray et al., 2022).

The first sign of erythema or macular, orange-red, scarlatiniform eruption can be inconspicuous and can be easily missed in darker-skinned babies leading to delayed diagnosis, more complications, and high mortality in an inexperienced setting. Extreme tenderness of the skin is an early feature in all skin types, and may occur at a stage at which cutaneous signs are not yet striking. The child is pyrexial and distressed. Within the next 24–48 hours the surface becomes wrinkled before starting to separate, leaving raw, red erosions. Sites of predilection are the central part of the face, the axillae, and the groins.

The rapid onset with marked cutaneous tenderness distinguishes it from most of the other causes of erythroderma in infancy. The main differential diagnosis is toxic epidermal necrolysis but TEN shows mucosal involvement.

Investigations

Mostly clinical diagnosis, but basic investigations are performed to assess liver, renal and haematological parameters, and blood cultures and antibiotic sensitivity (ABST).

Skin biopsy for histology is recommended; a frozen section provides rapid differentiation from TEN, when the level of split in TEN is lower at the subepidermal level, but is intraepidermal in SSSS.

Management

Treatment is with either a penicillinase-resistant penicillin analogue, such as co-amoxiclav, or with a cephalosporin; can adjust according to ABST. Heat and fluid losses and hyponatraemia should be dealt with. Pain will also require treatment, and affected infants will generally be much more comfortable if the lesions are dressed rather than left open (Leung et al., 2018).

Mortality is 2–10% in children with late diagnosis.

MYCOBACTERIAL

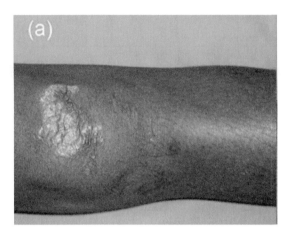

FIGURE 2.7A A 10-year-old boy came with a warty plaque on the left knee for more than 8 months that had been enlarging progressively. This was asymptomatic. He had no past history or contact history of pulmonary tuberculosis. He did not have a history of contact with fish or related hobbies. (Photographed by Dr. Ranthilaka R. Gammanpila.)

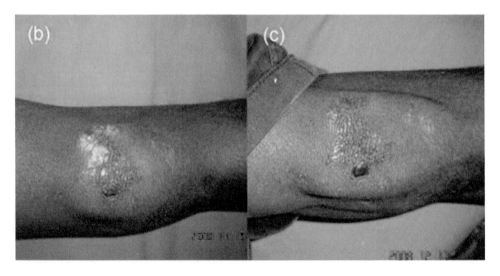

FIGURE 2.7B (b) After 3 months of anti-TB therapy. (c) After 4 months the lesion disappeared completely, but anti-TB therapy was continued for 6 months. (Photographed by Dr. Ranthilaka R. Gammanpila.)

Based on the clinical history and Figure 2.7a, what is your differential diagnosis?

1. Warty tuberculosis (tuberculous verrucosa cutis [TVC])
2. Fish tank granuloma
3. Viral wart

CUTANEOUS TUBERCULOSIS

Diagnosis

Warty tuberculosis (tuberculous verrucosa cutis [TVC])

Discussion

Causative organisms: *Mycobacterium tuberculosis*

Warty tuberculosis occurs by exogenous inoculation of bacteria in previously sensitized individuals. It can also occur by autoinoculation with sputum in a patient with active tuberculosis. The lesions are typically asymptomatic and start as a small, indurated, warty papule with a slight inflammatory areola.

This should be differentiated from other warty lesions such as fish tank granuloma (only distinguished by microbiological culture), viral wart, callosity, blastomycosis, chromoblastomycosis, actinomycosis, and leishmaniasis (Khandpur & Taneja, 2021)

Investigations

Skin biopsy will show granulomatous inflammation, but since the quantity of bacilli encountered in cutaneous lesions is small, stains for acid-fast bacilli are usually negative. Culture may be more helpful but positive in less than 12.5% of samples. PCR has been successfully used to confirm the diagnosis of lupus vulgaris. PCR positivity rates were 55% for tuberculosis verrucosa cutis (38 cases) and 60% for lupus vulgaris (5 cases) (Tan, 2001). Although positive results of ESR, Mantoux reactivity, and TB cultures facilitate the clinical diagnosis, negative results should not exclude the diagnosis of cutaneous TB (Ranawaka et al., 2010; Ranawaka, 2021a).

Management

Anti-TB treatment for six months.

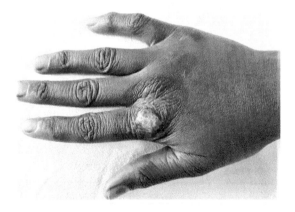

FIGURE 2.8 A 17-year-old boy came with a 4-week history of asymptomatic slow-growing pinkish plaque on his left dorsal hand. There was a history of accidental trauma while he was cleaning his fish tank about 2 months ago. (Photographed by Dr. Ajith P. Kannangara.)

Based on the clinical history and Figure 2.8, what is your differential diagnosis?

1. Fish tank granuloma
2. Tuberculoid leprosy
3. Chromoblastomycosis
4. Foreign body granuloma

FISH TANK GRANULOMA

Diagnosis

Fish tank granuloma

Discussion

Mycobacterium marinum infects fish and is often found in swimming pools, sea water, and fresh water. It is the most common nontuberculous mycobacterium to cause skin infection, which is often referred to as swimming pool granuloma or fish tank granuloma (Canetti et al., 2022).

The infection results from inoculation on the distal limb (e.g., accidental trauma to finger or hand) and induces a chronic wound, which fails to heal. After an incubation period of 2 to 3 weeks, solitary erythematous to violaceous, hyperkeratotic papules form. Subsequently these lesions develop into psoriasiform or verrucous nodules or plaques and tend to ulcerate. Multiple lesions may be present and extend proximally along sites of lymphatic drainage, in a sporotrichoid or lymphatic distribution. The lesions either spontaneously resolve in months or persist for years to heal with scarring. Lesions are usually limited to the skin because the organisms require a temperature of 30° to 32°C for optimal growth.

Investigations

The histological findings in *Mycobacterium marinum* infection vary and range from suppurative dermatitis with ulceration and necrosis in early lesions to tuberculoid granulomas at the late stage. The epidermis often shows hyperkeratosis and papillomatosis and is occasionally ulcerated. The early lesions may show AFB (Acid-Fast Bacillus) with Fite stain.

Management

Systemic dissemination is rare except for immunocompromised hosts. *Mycobacterium marinum* culture is often negative and the diagnosis is usually made clinically. Oral clarithromycin is usually effective for faster clearance; however, surgical debridement may be necessary for extensive cases (Pop et al., 2019).

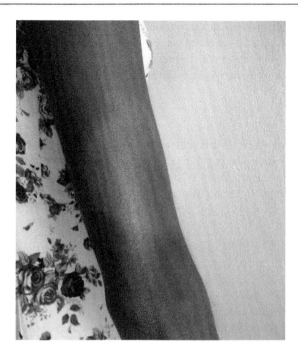

FIGURE 2.9 A 15-year-old girl came with a 4-month history of hypopigmented patch on her right arm and loss of sensation over the lesion subsequently. (Photographed by Dr. Ranthilaka R. Gammanpila.)

Based on the clinical history and Figure 2.9, what is your differential diagnosis?

1. Tuberculoid leprosy
2. Pityriasis versicolor
3. Naevus depigmentoses
4. Vitiligo

LEPROSY

Diagnosis

Tuberculoid leprosy

Discussion

In tuberculoid form of leprosy, only the nerves and skin show clinical evidence of disease. Lesions are few (one to five) conspicuous, erythematous, copper-coloured, or purple plaque, with raised and clear-cut edges sloping toward a flattened and hypopigmented centre. Erythema may be absent in dark-skinned people. The surface of the lesion is dry or scaly, insensitive, and hairless. Sensory impairment may be difficult to demonstrate due to generous sensory nerve supply of the face. Thickened sensory nerves can be palpated in nearby lesions. Some cases may be purely neural, with pain and swelling of the affected nerve followed by anesthesia and/or muscle weakness and wasting (Ranawaka, 2021b).

Investigations

Histopathological examination reveals tuberculoid granulomas collect in foci surrounding neurovascular elements. The granuloma invades the papillary zone and may even erode the epidermis, but AFB are not seen. Cutaneous nerves that are not destroyed appear greatly swollen by epithelioid cell granulomas and surrounded by a zone of lymphocytes; occasionally there may be caseation within the nerve.

Management

- Multidrug anti-leprosy treatment for leprosy is the stranded treatment with low relapse rates but needs to be taken over many months. According to 2018 WHO guidelines, all 3 drugs (clofizimine, rifampicin, and dapsone) are prescribed for 6 months for treatment of tuberculoid leprosy and 12 months for multibacillary leprosy.
- **For children 10-14 years:** Rifampicin 450 mg once a month, clofazimine 150 mg once a month and 50 mg on alternate days, and dapsone 50 mg daily is recommended, 12 months for MB leprosy and 6 months for PB leprosy.
- **For children (<10 years old or <40kg):** Rifampicin 10 mg/kg once a month, clofazimine 100 mg once a month and 50 mg twice weekly, and dapsone 2 mg/kg daily is recommended, 12 months for MB leprosy and 6 months for PB leprosy (WHO, 2018).

VIRAL

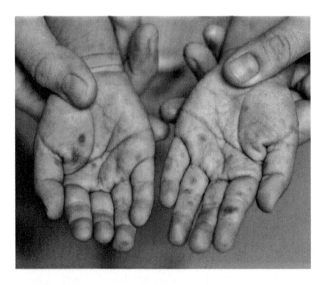

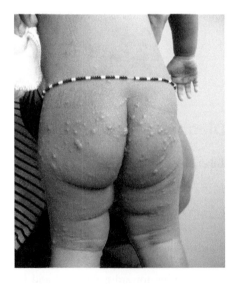

FIGURE 2.10A   A 3-year-old boy was directed to the skin clinic by a paediatrician, with blistering eruptions mainly on palms and soles and a few mouth lesions. (Photographed by Dr. Ajith P. Kannangara.)

FIGURE 2.10B Asymptomatic vesicular eruption on knees and buttocks in a 5-month-old baby. (Photographed by Dr. Ranthilaka R. Gammanpila.)

Based on the clinical history and Figure 2.10a, what is your differential diagnosis?

1. Hand foot and mouth disease
2. Herpangina
3. Erythema multiforme

HAND FOOT AND MOUTH DISEASE

Diagnosis

Hand foot and mouth disease

Discussion

Hand foot and mouth disease is a contagious dermatosis caused by enteroviruses, most commonly Coxsackie virus A16 and enterovirus 71. Transmission appears mainly through respiratory droplets and sometimes the faecal–oral route. It predominantly affects children under 5 years old (Peng et al., 2023). Eruption is characterized by the presence of an oral enanthem and papular-vesicular rash on the palms, soles, face, and buttocks. Mucosal lesions appear as small vesicles on the buccal mucosa, hard palate, and tongue, and evolve to small, painful ulcers with erythematous halo. Cutaneous vesicular lesions become covered by a crust and heal without scarring. Patients may present fever, cough, sore mouth, and loss of appetite (Rajendiran, 2021).

Investigations

This is mainly a clinical diagnosis.

Management

Symptomatic management only; in severe infection, oral acyclovir is prescribed for one week.

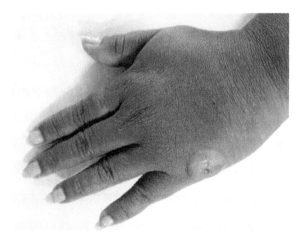

FIGURE 2.11   An 18-year-girl from a rural village presented with 3 days' history of painful exudative bullous lesion on her left dorsal hand. There was a history of helping her father who is a farmer with handling domestic cows during the milking process. (Photographed by Dr. Ajith P. Kannangara.)

Based on the clinical history and Figure 2.11, what is your differential diagnosis?

1. Milker's nodule
2. Atypical mycobacteriosis
3. Orf (Ecthyma contagiosum)

MILKER'S NODULE (PSEUDO COWPOX OR PARA VACCINIA)

Diagnosis

Milker's nodule (Pseudo cowpox or Para vaccinia)

Discussion

Milker's nodule, also known as Para vaccinia and pseudo cowpox, is an occupational disease caused by the Para vaccinia virus, a Parapox virus. The virus is transmitted mainly from infected cattle, by contact with the animals or contaminated objects. Human-to-human transmission is not common. It affects milkers, veterinarians, or persons who handle fresh meat. Incubation period usually varies between 5 and 15 days.

Clinical aspect is like Orf (ecthyma contagiosum). One or a few lesions appear on the exposed sites (hands, forearms, and face). At the onset, they present as erythematous maculopapular lesions which evolve in six stages including maculopapular, target-oid, nodular, exudative, regenerative, and regressive. Cutaneous lesions may be associated with pain, regional lymph node enlargement, or secondary bacterial infection (Fox et al., 2023).

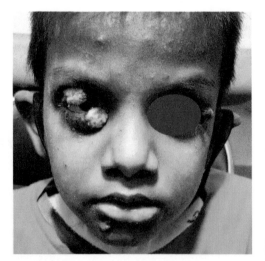

Investigations

Histopathological examination reveals keratinocytes with eosinophilic inclusions and electron microscopy shows characteristic brick-shaped viral particles.

Management

This is a self-limiting condition. Treatment is supportive, including antiseptics, analgesics, and antibiotics. Cutaneous lesions heal without scarring. Infection creates lasting immunity for the patient affected.

FIGURE 2.12A A 7-year-old boy came with 2-month history of giant warty lesions on his face. (Photographed by Dr. Ajith P. Kannangara.)

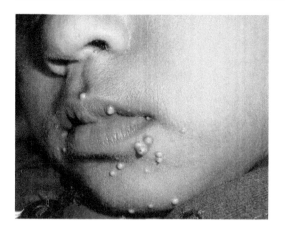

FIGURE 2.12B Molluscum contagiosum in a 7-month-old infant. (Photographed by Dr. Ranthilaka R. Gammanpila.)

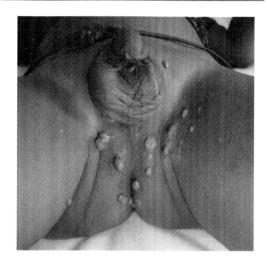

FIGURE 2.12C A 2-year-old boy with molluscum contagiosum in perineal skin. (Photographed by Dr. Ranthilaka R. Gammanpila.)

Based on the clinical history and Figure 2.12a, what is your differential diagnosis?

1. Molluscum contagiosum
2. Verruca vulgaris
3. Eruptive xanthomas
4. Keratoacanthoma

MOLLUSCUM CONTAGIOSUM

Diagnosis

Molluscum contagiosum

Discussion

Molluscum contagiosum is a viral infection of the skin and mucous membranes caused by a poxvirus. It is frequently found in children with lesions on the face, torso, and hands and in young adults with lesions on the breasts, thighs, and genital area. In children, the virus is transmitted through direct contact with infected persons. Clinically one or multiple lesions represented by firm, small papules (2–5 mm in diameter), flesh-coloured with smooth surfaces and central umbilication can appear. Sometimes they may be associated with pruritus, erythema, and bacterial superinfection. Scratching may cause viral spread through autoinoculation. In immunocompromised patients, lesions are more numerous and extremely large.

Investigations

This is usually a clinical diagnosis, sometimes needing histopathological examination.

Management

Lesions may persist from months to years. Treatment options include curettage, cryotherapy, imiquimod, podophyllin, dilute povidone-iodine, intralesional 5-fluorouracil, or electrocoagulation.

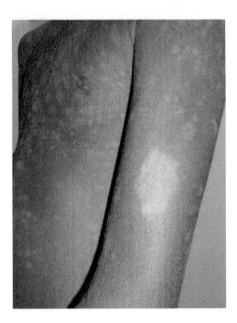 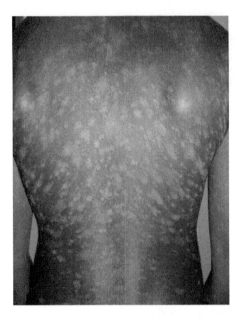

FIGURE 2.13A, 2.13B   An 11-year-old boy presented with this asymptomatic generalized rash on the trunk and limbs. Note the more prominent (the largest) lesion, which appeared first on his left arm. (Photographed by Dr. Ranthilaka R. Gammanpila.)

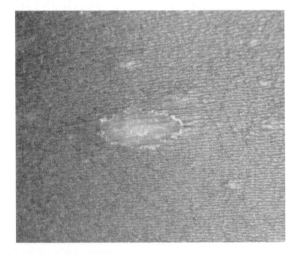

FIGURE 2.13C   A sharply defined, erythematous, round or oval macule, centre tending to clear, with a marginal collarette of scale. (Photographed by Dr. Ranthilaka R. Gammanpila.)

Based on the clinical history and Figure 2.13, what is your differential diagnosis?

1. Pityriasis rosea
2. Viral exanthum
3. Drug rash

PITYRIASIS ROSEA

Diagnosis

Pityriasis rosea

Discussion

Pityriasis rosea is acute self-limiting disease with possible viral aetiology. A pityriasis rosea-like reaction has been reported for several drugs. It is common in the 10-to-35-years' age group; uncommon in infancy and old age.

The "herald patch", which appears first, is larger and more conspicuous (Figure 2.13a). P. rosea lesions are sharply defined, erythematous, round or oval macule, centre tending to clear, with a marginal collarette of scale attached peripherally, with the free edge of the scale internally (Figure 2.13c). After an interval, which is usually between 5 and 15 days, the general eruption begins to appear in crops over few weeks. The long axes of the lesions characteristically follow the lines of cleavage parallel to the ribs in a Christmas tree pattern on the upper chest and back (Figure 2.13b). Except for mild pruritus, it is mostly asymptomatic. These self-limit over 2–3 months without any residual effects.

Pityriasis rosea may be atypical in appearance, distribution of the lesions, or in its course: absent herald patch, more generalized, limited to a few lesions often around the herald patch, papular or urticarial eruption, etc.

Investigations

This is a clinical diagnosis.

Management

Symptomatic treatment. Educate the parents on self-limiting nature.

If itch is troublesome, or the appearance distressing, a topical steroid, usually of moderate potency or UVB, can be helpful.

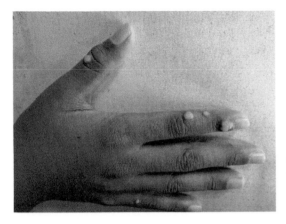

FIGURE 2.14A A 13-year-old girl came with multiple warty lesions on hands. (Photographed by Dr. Ranthilaka R. Gammanpila.)

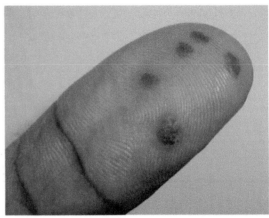

FIGURE 2.14B Palmar warts.

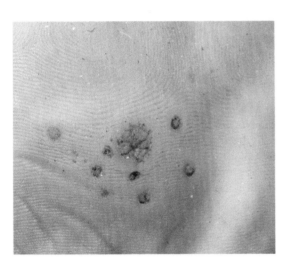

FIGURE 2.14C Mosaic plantar warts.

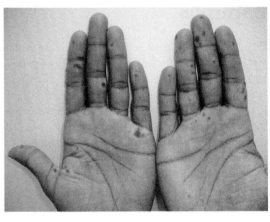

FIGURE 2.14D Multiple palmar warts. (Photographed by Dr. Ranthilaka R. Gammanpila.)

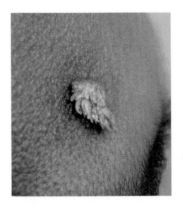

FIGURE 2.14E Filiform or digitate wart.

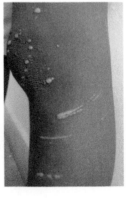

FIGURE 2.14F Koebner phenomenon.

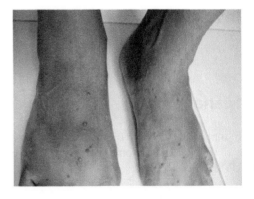

FIGURE 2.14G Plane warts. (Photographed by Dr. Ranthilaka R. Gammanpila.)

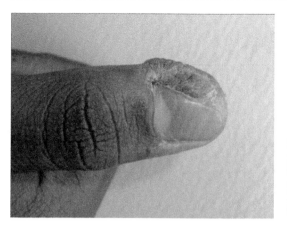

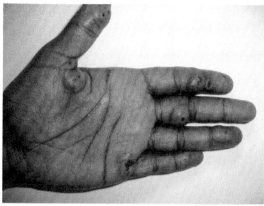

FIGURE 2.14H Periungual warts. (Photographed by Dr. Ranthilaka R. Gammanpila.)

FIGURE 2.14I Blistering following liquid nitrogen cryotherapy. This is a well-known cutaneous reaction which may be managed with oral antibiotics, topical antibiotics, and pain killers. (Photographed by Dr. Ranthilaka R. Gammanpila.)

Based on the clinical history and Figure 2.14a, what is your diagnosis?

1. Common warts (verruca vulgaris)
2. Plane warts (verruca plana)

VIRAL WARTS

Diagnosis

Common warts (verruca vulgaris)

Discussion

Human papillomavirus (HPV) infection.

Warts on the skin may present in a number of different morphological forms, dependent on virus type, body site, immunological status of the patient, and environmental influences: 70% common warts, 24% plantar warts, 3.5% plane warts, 2.0% filiform warts, 0.5% ano-genital warts and periungual warts. New warts may form at sites of trauma due to the Koebner-like isomorphic phenomenon.

Plane warts are smooth, flat, or slightly elevated, usually skin-coloured or greyish yellow, but may be pigmented. They are round or polygonal in shape and vary in size from 1 to 5 mm.

Management

Spontaneous clearance of warts can occur at any time from a few months to years. The 16–40% salicylic acid lotion or creams, liquid nitrogen cryotherapy are widely used to treat. Topical podophyllotoxin, imiquimod or cryotherapy are used for ano-genital warts.

FUNGAL

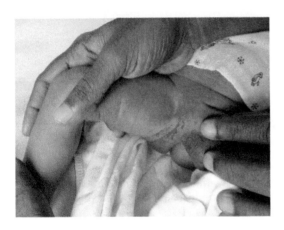

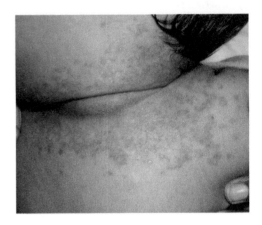

FIGURE 2.15A A 2-week-old neonate had this lesion on groins and perianal area. This was asymptomatic and was an incidental finding. (Photographed by Dr. Ranthilaka R. Gammanpila.)

FIGURE 2.15B Candida intertrigo in a 3-month-old obese baby. Note the deep red colour and moisture in the folds and satellite lesions at the periphery. (Photographed by Dr. Ranthilaka R. Gammanpila.)

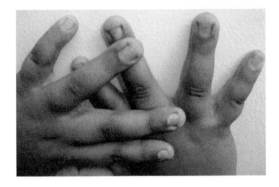

FIGURE 2.15C Candida intertrigo on web spaces in a 3-year-old boy. Finger web or toe web candidosis is uncommon in younger children, and detailed inquiry into this child revealed OCD washing of hands 20–30 times per day. (Photographed by Dr. Ranthilaka R. Gammanpila.)

Based on the clinical history and Figure 2.15a, what is your differential diagnosis?

1. Candida intertrigo
2. Irritant contact dermatitis
3. Napkin dermatitis

CANDIDA INTERTRIGO

Diagnosis

Candida intertrigo or flexural candidosis

Discussion

Erythema with a moist exudation starts in the deep folds. Then the typical features of candidosis develop with a fringed, irregular edge and subcorneal pustules rupturing to give tiny erosions. Satellite lesions, pustular or papular, are classic. Intense soreness and itching are usual in older children and in adults.

Investigations

This is a clinical diagnosis.

Management

- Topical antifungal creams, azole, or polyene creams for about 2 weeks cure the lesions completely. In obese babies applying antifungal powders to skin creases may prevent recurrent candida growth. Attention should be given to keep the affected area dry; potassium permanganate soaks are effective in some.
- Oral candidosis is treated with clotrimazole or miconazole oral gels.
- If the predisposing factors are found as in obsessive compulsive disorder (OCD), that should be dealt with.

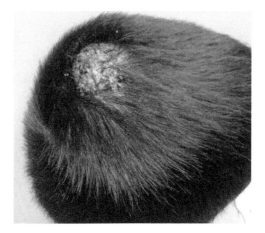

FIGURE 2.16   A 5-year-old boy was brought with a rapidly developing boggy mass on the scalp for 5 days in spite of the antibiotics prescribed by their family physician. The child was clinically well. (Photographed by Dr. Ranthilaka R. Gammanpila.)

Based on the clinical history and Figure 2.16, what is your differential diagnosis?

1. Kerion
2. Abscess

KERION

Diagnosis

Kerion

Discussion

The most severe pattern of tinea capitis is known as kerion. It is a painful, inflammatory mass, and thick crusting with matting of adjacent hairs is common. Caused by one of the zoophilic species, typically *T. verrucosum* or *T. mentagrophytes*.

Patients present with rapidly enlarging boggy mass on the scalp in spite of oral antibiotics. The children are clinically well and afebrile that is non-corresponding to the inflammatory mass. Lymphadenopathy is frequent. If treatment is delayed, permanent hair loss from scarring is usual (Ranawaka, 2021c).

Management

- The careful removal of crusts using wet compresses is important.
- Coexisting bacterial infection should be treated.
- Duration of oral antifungal therapy is assessed clinically, depending on the clinical response, which should be continued until total clearance of the infection and inflammation.

  - Terbinafine: <10 kg, 62.5 mg; 10–20 kg, 125 mg; >20 kg, 250 mg
  - Itraconazole 2–4 mg/kg/day
  - Griseofulvin 10 mg/kg (20 mg/kg considered in some)
  - Permanent hair loss from scarring can be prevented by early onset of treatments.

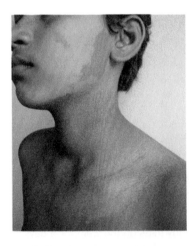

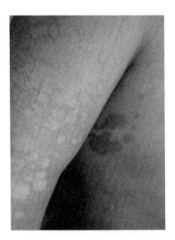

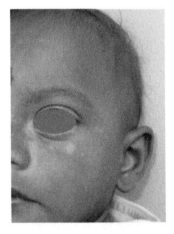

FIGURE 2.17A A 13-year-old boy came with mildly itchy (especially after outdoor playing) hypopigmented macular lesion over the chest for more than 6 months. (Photographed by Dr. Ranthilaka R. Gammanpila.)

FIGS. 2.17B Hypopigmented and hyperpigmented pityriasis versicolor in the same person. (Photographed by Dr. Ranthilaka R. Gammanpila.)

FIGURE 2.17C In infants pityriasis versicolor is common around the eyes (periorbital.) (Photographed by Dr. Ranthilaka R. Gammanpila.)

Based on the clinical history and Figure 2.17a, what is your differential diagnosis?

1. Pityriasis versicolor
2. Vitiligo
3. Pityriasis alba
4. Indeterminate
5. Post inflammatory hypopigmentation

PITYRIASIS VERSICOLOR

Diagnosis

Pityriasis versicolor

Discussion

Pityriasis versicolor, also called tinea versicolor, is a mild, chronic, superficial fungal infection of the stratum corneum, characterized by scaly, dyspigmented irregular macules most often occurring on the trunk and extremities. Its skin lesions are characterized by well-demarcated macules, with slight desquamation and colour ranging from white to brownish and brown. The involved skin regions are usually the trunk, back, abdomen, face, and proximal extremities. Hypopigmented lesions often arise in patients with a dark skin phototype after exposure to the sun. Usually, hyperpigmented skin patches give the affected area a darker-than-normal skin colour. Involvement of the scalp and genitalia are less common. In children, it is characterized by depigmented lesions that usually affect the face, and specifically the forehead, in contrast to adult presentations.

Investigations

Diagnosis is mainly clinical. Skin scraping for fungal study, Wood's lamp examination and dermatoscopy may be helpful to exclude differential diagnoses.

Management

Topical antifungal therapy is generally sufficient. In a case of widespread disease, ketoconazole, itraconazole, or fluconazole are administered. Since tinea versicolor may be recurrent, preventive measures should be taken.

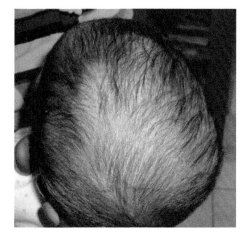

FIGURE 2.18A A 3-month-old baby was brought complaining of itchy scaly scalp. On examination, a well-demarcated finely scaly area was noted. In this child the inflammation is minimal, but fine scaling is characteristic, with a fairly sharp margin. (Photographed by Dr. Ranthilaka R. Gammanpila.)

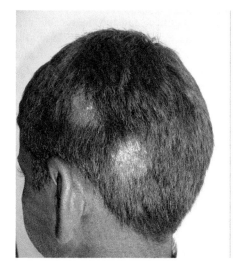

FIGURE 2.18B Tinea capitis in a 6-year-old boy. Well-circumscribed areas of itchy, scaly, patchy hair loss with evidence of inflammation. (Photographed by Dr. Ranthilaka R. Gammanpila.)

Based on the clinical history and Figure 2.18a, what is your differential diagnosis?

1. Tinea capitis
2. Dandruff
3. Cradle cap

TINEA CAPITIS

Diagnosis

Tinea capitis

Discussion

This is ringworm of the scalp caused by invasion of the hair shafts by a dermatophyte fungus; *Microsporum canis* and *Trychophyton tonsurans* are the commonest causative fungi. Tinea capitis predominantly affects children.

There are three types depending on the hair invasion by the fungi: ectothrix, endothrix, and favus (Hay & Ashbee, 2016).

Ectothrix type is caused by *Microsporum species*, especially *M. audouinii*. Fluorescence under Wood's lamp is characteristically present in this type of hair invasion.

Endothrix type may be caused by *Trichophyton species*. Affected hair is fragile, and breaks off close to the scalp surface. This type is non-fluorescent.

Favus, or favic type, is caused by *T. schoenleinii*. The affected hair is less damaged than in other types, and may continue to grow. Greenish grey fluorescence is present.

The clinical appearance of tinea capitis varies depending on the type of hair invasion, the level of host resistance, and the degree of inflammatory host response. This can vary from a few dull grey, broken-off hairs with a little scaling, detectable only on careful inspection (Figure 2.18a), marked single or multiple patches of alopecia (Figure 2.18b) to a severe, painful, inflammatory mass (kerion) (Figure 2.16). In all types, the cardinal features are partial hair loss with inflammation of some degree.

Management

Anti-fungal shampoos with creams are sufficient in small children.

Older children and extensive patches are treated with oral antifungals in addition to topical shampoos and creams.

- Terbinafine: <10 kg, 62.5 mg; 10–20 kg, 125 mg; >20 kg, 250 mg; all given daily for 4 weeks
- Itraconazole 2–4 mg/kg/day for 4–6 weeks
- Griseofulvin 10 mg/kg for 6 weeks (20 mg/kg considered in some *T. tonsurans* and *T. schoenleinii* infections)

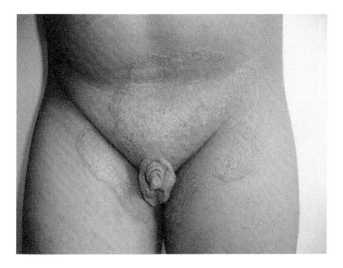

FIGURE 2.19 A 2-year-old boy came with itchy annular scaly lesions on his trunk and perineum for one month. (Photographed by Dr. Ranthilaka R. Gammanpila.)

Based on the clinical history and Figure 2.19, what is your differential diagnosis?

1. Tinea infection
2. Subacute cutaneous lupus erythematosus (SCLE)
3. Nummular eczema
4. Psoriasis
5. Pityriasis rosea

TINEA CORPORIS

Diagnosis

Tinea infection

Discussion

Tinea is a cutaneous dermatophyte skin infection occurring in sites other the feet, groin, face, or hand. Common organisms are *T. rubrum*, *T. tonsurans*, and *M. canis*. Typically, the lesion begins as an erythematous, scaly plaque with a slightly elevated edge that may rapidly worsen and enlarge. The central area becomes brown or hypopigmented and less scaly as the active border progresses outward.

Management

Tinea corporis is normally treated by topical agents such as allylamines, ciclopirox, and amorolfine. In a case of widespread or recalcitrant tinea cruris, oral antifungal drugs should be considered.

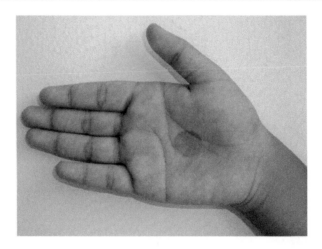

FIGURE 2.20   A 6-year-old boy presented with asymptomatic hyperpigmented circular patch on his right palm for more than 3 months. It had been gradually enlarging in size. (Photographed by Dr. Ranthilaka R. Gammanpila.)

Based on the clinical history and Figure 2.20, what is your differential diagnosis?

1. Tinea nigra
2. Tinea manuum
3. Acquired melanocytic naevus

TINEA NIGRA

Diagnosis

Tinea nigra

Discussion

Tinea nigra is an asymptomatic, superficial fungal infection caused by *Hortaea werneckii*. This is more common in tropical climates. The lesions are asymptomatic; they are macular, sharply defined and not scaly; the most distinctive feature is the brown or black colour. The palms are most commonly affected, but other areas of the body such as the soles, neck, and trunk have been reported.

Investigations

This is a clinical diagnosis. Microscopy of infected epidermal scales in potassium hydroxide (KOH) and/or culture will isolate the fungi.

Management

Topical azole creams such as econazole and ketoconazole are recommended until complete clearance is achieved.

PARASITIC

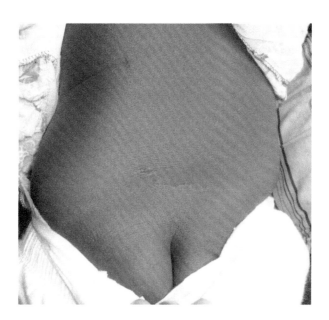

FIGURE 2.21 A 5-month-old baby was brought with this linear itchy lesion for 2 days. Parents have noticed that this lesion is moving forward. (Photographed by Dr. Ranthilaka R. Gammanpila.)

Based on the clinical history and Figure 2.21, what is your differential diagnosis?

1. Cutaneous larva migrans or creeping eruption
2. Larva currens ("running larva") of strongyloidiasis
3. Migratory myiasis

CUTANEOUS LARVA MIGRANS

Diagnosis

Cutaneous larva migrans

Discussion

The prime feature here is the creeping or migrating lesion/s, and that they are due to the presence of moving parasites in the skin.

Causative organisms are:

- *Ancylostoma brasiliense* (dog and cat hookworm)
- *Ancylostoma caninum* (dog hookworm)

- *Ancylostoma ceylonicum*
- *Unicararia stenocephala* (dog hookworm)
- *Bubostumum phlebotomum* (cattle hookworm)

These are all hookworms of various animals; the dog hookworm is the commonest cause of creeping eruption in humans. Adult hookworms live in the intestines of dogs and cats, and their ova are deposited in the animals' faeces. Under favourable conditions of humidity and temperature, the ova hatch into infective larvae, which will penetrate human skin. This is commonly the feet, hands, and buttocks. When they creep, exceedingly itchy, slightly raised, flesh-coloured or pink, bizarre, serpentine patterns are formed. The cutaneous lesions only progress a few millimetres to a few centimetres daily.

The main distinguishing factor to differentiate larvae currens is the speed at which the larvae travel; 5–15 cm/h.

Investigations

This is a clinical diagnosis.

Management

The disease is self-limiting, and may last for weeks or months if untreated.

- Ivermectin 200 µg/kg orally once daily for 1 or 2 days
- Albendazole 400 mg orally for 3 days

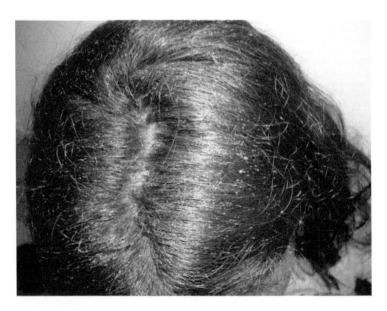

FIGURE 2.22 A 12-year-old girl came with an infected, badly smelly scalp. On inspection of the scalp numerous nits were detected. (Photographed by Dr. Ranthilaka R. Gammanpila.)

Based on the clinical history and Figure 2.22, what is your differential diagnosis?

1. Pediculus capitis and secondary bacterial infection on scalp
2. Dandruff and secondary bacterial infection on scalp

PEDICULOSIS

Diagnosis

Pediculus capitis (head lice)

Discussion

Head louse infestation (pediculosis capitis) is common both in developed and developing countries. This is more common on girls, particularly in the age range 3–11 years. Head-to-head contact is frequent in these age groups and favours the spread. Older children tend to be more independent, and more separated from their peers.

Scalp pruritus is the characteristic manifestation of head louse infection. Secondary bacterial infection may occur as a result of scratching.

Management

The ideal treatment should be completely safe, free of harmful chemicals, readily available, easy to use, and inexpensive.(Monsel, 2016)

Permethrin and pyrethroid insecticides are widely used today. Advise to repeat treatment after 7–10 days because of limited ovicidal activity. Lotion and liquid formulations are preferable to shampoos because the latter expose the insects to relatively low concentrations of insecticide. Family members should be examined, and treated only if they show evidence of active infestation by the presence of live lice. Nits may be removed with a fine-toothed comb. All affected individuals in the household are treated simultaneously. All materials that touched the heads of infested persons, such as hats, scarves, bedding, and cushions, must be thoroughly washed in hot water (50°C at least).

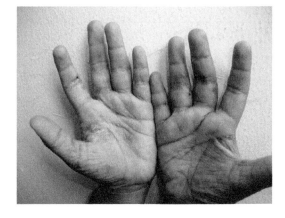

FIGURE 2.23A   A 5-year-old child came with generalized itchiness for one week. Itchiness was worse during the night, and his 10-month-old brother also had a similar problem. (Photographed by Dr. Ranthilaka R. Gammanpila.)

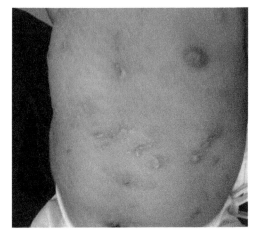

FIGURE 2.23B   Note burrows in this infant. (Photographed by Dr. Ranthilaka R. Gammanpila.)

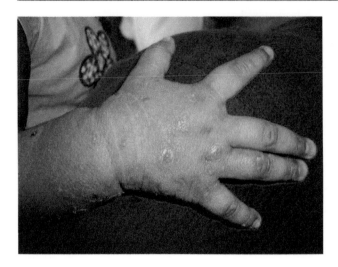

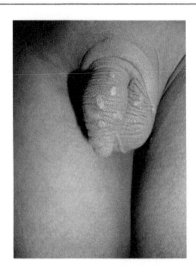

FIGURE 2.23C Itchy pustules and papules on finger webs and genitalia are the commonest clinical presentation in scabies. (Photographed by Dr. Ranthilaka R. Gammanpila.)

FIGURE 2.23D Scabitic nodules on genitals in a boy. Very itchy papules on male genitalia are characteristic of scabies and are resistant to therapy. (Photographed by Dr. Ranthilaka R. Gammanpila.)

Based on the clinical history and Figure 2.23a, what is your differential diagnosis?

1. Scabies
2. Infected eczema
3. Papular urticaria
4. Acute urticaria

SCABIES

Diagnosis

Scabies

Discussion

Scabies is an ectoparasitic infection caused in humans by the *Sarcoptes scabiei* var. *hominis*. Copulation occurs in a small burrow excavated by the female. Approximately 40–50 eggs are laid by each female during a lifespan of 4–6 weeks. Eggs hatch after 3–4 days into larvae, which dig new burrows closer to the skin surface. There, the larvae mature into adult mites in about 4 days (Monsel et al., 2016).

Itching is the most obvious manifestation of scabies, usually sparing the face in adult classic scabies. It is generally worse at night when the patient is warm. Typical locations of lesions are the finger webs, the flexor surfaces of the wrists, the elbows, the axillae, the buttocks, and the genitalia. The typical lesions of scabies are burrows, which appear as slightly raised brownish tortuous lesions. Inflammatory pruritic papules or nodules, sometimes surmounted by burrows, on the male genitalia are characteristic (Gunasekara, 2021).

Investigations

The presence of genital lesions in men or breast nodules in women is strongly suggestive. Absolute confirmation can only be made by the discovery of burrows and/or microscopic examination. A burrow is gently scraped off the skin with a blunt scalpel, and the material placed in mineral oil on a microscope slide. The presence of mites, eggs, fragments of egg shells, or scybala confirms the diagnosis. Failure to find mites is common and does not rule out scabies.

Management

Treatment should be prescribed to the patient and close physical contacts, even without pruritus or cutaneous lesions.

- Benzyl benzoate, esdepallethrine, and permethrin may be used in infants.
- Benzyl benzoate and esdepallethrine are safe in children <2 years of age, but duration of use should be limited to 12 h.
- Ivermectin is contraindicated in children <15 kg.

Treating the face of babies is essential because transmission may occur by breastfeeding. All clothes and bedding must be washed at high temperature (>50°C) or must be kept in a plastic bag for up to 72 h. Itching may persist several weeks after scabies, and this should be clearly explained to the parents.

REFERENCES

Canetti D, Riccardi N, Antonello RM, Nozza S, Sotgiu G (2022). Mycobacterium marinum: A brief update for clinical purposes. *The European Journal of Internal Medicine*;105:15–9. doi: 10.1016/j.ejim.2022.07.013. Epub 2022 Jul 19.

Forouzan P, Cohen PR (2020). Erythrasma revisited: Diagnosis, differential diagnoses, and comprehensive review of treatment. *Cureus* 30;12(9):e10733. doi: 10.7759/cureus.10733.

Fox T, Gould S, Princy N, et al (2023). Therapeutics for treating mpox in humans. *Cochrane Database Systematic Reviews* 14;3(3):CD015769. doi: 10.1002/14651858.CD015769.

Gray L, Olson J, Brintz BJ, Cipriano SD (2022). Staphylococcal scalded skin syndrome: Clinical features, ancillary testing, and patient management. *Pediatric Dermatology*;39(6):908–913. doi: 10.1111/pde.15102. Epub 2022 Aug 16.

Gunasekara H (2021). Diseases caused by arthropods and parasites (2021). In Ranawaka RR, Kannangara AP, Karawita, A, eds. *Atlas of Dermatoses in Pigmented Skin*. Singapore: Springer, pp. 397–416.

Hay RJ, Ashbee HR (2016). Fungal infections. In Christopher G, Jonathan B, Tanya B, Robert C, Daniel C, eds. *Rook's Textbook of Dermatology*, 9th edn. Hoboken: Wiley-Blackwell, 32.1p.

Khandpur S, Taneja N (2021). Cutaneous tuberculosis. In: Ranawaka RR, Kannangara AP, Karawita, A, eds. *Atlas of Dermatoses in Pigmented Skin*. Singapore: Springer, pp. 227–36.

Leung AKC, Barankin B, Leong KF (2018). Staphylococcal-scalded skin syndrome: Evaluation, diagnosis, and management. *World Journal of Pediatrics*;14(2):116–20. doi: 10.1007/s12519-018-0150-x. Epub 2018 Mar 5.

Monsel G, Delaunay P, Chosidow O (2016). Arthropods. In Christopher G, Jonathan B, Tanya B, Robert C, Daniel C, eds. *Rook's Textbook of Dermatology*, 9th edn. Hoboken: Wiley-Blackwell, 34.18p.

Ongsri P, LeeyaPhan C, Limphoka P, KiRatiwongwan R, Bunyaratavej S (2021). Effectiveness and safety of zinc oxide nanoparticle-coated socks compared to uncoated socks for the prevention of pitted keratolysis: A double-blinded, randomized, controlled trial study. *The International Journal of Dermatology*;60(7):864–7. doi: 10.1111/ijd.15512. Epub 2021 Mar 4.

Pattanaprichakul P, Kulthanan K, Bunyaratavej S, et al. (2021) The Correlations between clinical features, dermoscopic and histopathological findings, and treatment outcomes of patients with pitted keratolysis. *BioMed Research International* 25;2021:3416643. doi: 10.1155/2021/3416643.

Peng Y, He W, Zheng Z, et al (2023). Factors related to the mortality risk of severe hand, foot, and mouth diseases (HFMD): A 5-year hospital-based survey in Guangxi, Southern China. *BMC Infectious Diseases* 8;23(1):144. doi: 10.1186/s12879-023-08109-y.

Pop R, Estermann L, Schulthess B, Eberhard N (2019). Deep infection with *Mycobacterium marinum*: successful treatment of a frequently misdiagnosed disease. *BMJ Case Reports* 28;12(8):e229663. doi: 10.1136/bcr-2019-229663.

Rajendiran P (2021). Viral infections. In Ranawaka RR, Kannangara AP, Karawita, A, eds. *Atlas of Dermatoses in Pigmented Skin*. Singapore: Springer, pp. 297–318.

Ranawaka RR (2021a). Mycobacterial infections in Sri Lanka. In Ranawaka RR, Kannangara AP, Karawita, A, eds. *Atlas of Dermatoses in Pigmented Skin*. Singapore: Springer, pp. 237–56.

Ranawaka RR (2021b). Leprosy. In Ranawaka RR, Kannangara AP, Karawita, A, eds. *Atlas of Dermatoses in Pigmented Skin*. Singapore: Springer, pp. 257–96.

Ranawaka RR (2021c). Superficial fungal infections. In Ranawaka RR, Kannangara AP, Karawita, A, eds. *Atlas of Dermatoses in Pigmented Skin*. Singapore: Springer, pp. 319–58

Ranawaka RR, AbEygunasekara PH, Perera E, Weerakoon HS (2010). Clinico-histopathological correlation and the treatment response of 20 patients with cutaneous tuberculosis. *The Dermatology Online Journal*;16(8):13.

Shrestha R, Karki S, Khadka M, Sapkota S, Timilsina B, Khadka S (2023). Meningococcemia in an 11 months old infant. *Case Reports in Infectious Diseases* 8;2023:8951318. doi: 10.1155/2023/8951318.

Tan SH, Tan HH, Sun YJ, Goh CL (2001). Clinical utility of polymerase chain reaction in the detection of Mycobacterium tuberculosis in different types of cutaneous tuberculosis and tuberculids. *Annals, Academy of Medicine, Singapore*;30(1):3–10.

World Health Organization. Regional Office for South-East Asia. (2018). Guidelines for the diagnosis, treatment and prevention of leprosy. World Health Organization. Regional Office for South-East Asia. https://apps.who.int/iris/handle/10665/274127.

Eczema, Dermatitis, and Ichthyosis in Children with FST 5

3

Ranthilaka R. Gammanpila

INTRODUCTION

This chapter discusses eczemas and dermatitis in children with brown skin (Fitzpatrick skin type V/FST 5). These are discussed based on clinical photographs and easy-to-read question and answer format. Most of these skin problems leave a post inflammatory hypopigmentation that is very common in darker-skinned infants and children that may arouse parental anxiety of vitiligo.

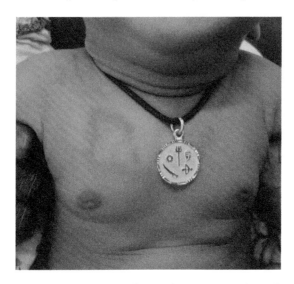

FIGURE 3.1 A 3-month-old child came with an itchy, erythematous patch on the chest for one month.

Based on the case description and Figure 3.1, what are your differential diagnoses?

1. Allergic contact dermatitis to the pendant
2. Infantile seborrhoeic dermatitis
3. Atopic eczema

DOI: 10.1201/9781003321507-3

ALLERGIC CONTACT DERMATITIS

Diagnosis

Allergic contact dermatitis

Discussion

To identify the possible contact allergen, the knowledge of one's culture, customs, clothing, food and living conditions is important. Giving bronze or gold pendants to babies is a custom in Asian countries (Srisaravanapavananthan, 2021). Erythema around the neck and erythema limited to the skin area touching the pendant is a clue to the diagnosis (Ranawaka, 2021a).

Investigations

This is a clinical diagnosis. Patch testing using suspected allergens can confirm the clinical diagnosis, but it is not routinely performed in children.

Management

Educate the parents on the possible causative factor/s. Advise them to remove the allergen. Mild topical steroid would relieve the symptoms.

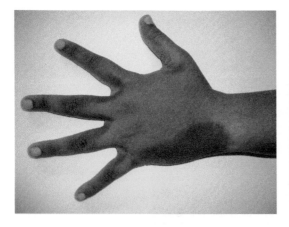 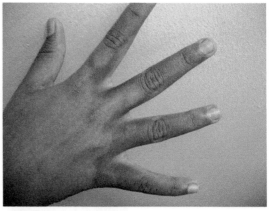

FIGURE 3.2A A 9-year-old girl came with these hyperpigmented patches on the dorsum of her hand, and interdigital areas. These have appeared overnight. Direct inquiry revealed that she had squeezed lime juice on the previous day.

FIGURES 3.2B Note the bizarrely shaped hyperpigmentation on sun-exposed areas. Direct inquiry revealed squeezing citrus fruits 2 days before the skin rash.

Based on the case description and Figure 3.2a, what are your differential diagnoses?

1. Post-inflammatory hyperpigmentation
2. Berloque dermatitis-like skin reaction
3. Phytophotodermatitis

BERLOQUE DERMATITIS

Diagnosis

Berloque dermatitis

Discussion

Berloque dermatitis-like skin reaction is common among our children, who have a history of squeezing lime or other citrus fruits such as oranges or lemons, and exposing to sunlight. Within 24 hours of contact with citrus juice they get this asymptomatic bizarrely shaped hyperpigmentation corresponding to the contact area; finger webs are common.

Berloque dermatitis is a type of photocontact dermatitis. This was first described after perfumed products containing bergamot (or a psoralen) are applied to the skin followed by exposure to sunlight. Striking linear patterns of hyperpigmentation are characteristic, corresponding to local application of the scented product. Berloque dermatitis results from the potentiation of UV-stimulated melanogenesis by 5-methoxypsoralen (bergapten) in perfumes containing bergamot oil (van Geel & Speeckaert, 2016).

Investigations

This is a clinical diagnosis.

Management

Reassurance only: usually this pigmentation fades away spontaneously after few weeks. Sometimes this may persist for months.

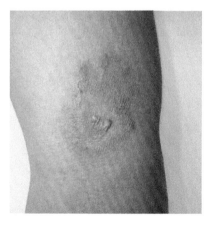

FIGURE 3.3 This 6-year-old village child who lives close to a paddy field developed this lesion overnight. The lesion was itchy with a burning sensation. He had been getting new lesions 2–3 days per week for last 2 months. The parents noticed similar lesions on his 3-year-old sister, too.

Based on the case description and Figure 3.3, what are your differential diagnoses?

1. Blister beetle dermatitis
2. Irritant contact dermatitis
3. "Witch spell"

BLISTER BEETLE DERMATITIS

Diagnosis

Blister beetle dermatitis

Discussion

Blister beetle dermatitis is an irritant contact dermatitis to the toxins released by blister beetles (*Paederus brasilensis*). The vesicant chemical in the body fluids of these insects causes an acute irritant contact dermatitis characterized by erythemato-vesicular lesions associated with a burning sensation on exposed parts of the body (Srihari et al., 2017). The patients give a history of burning and itchy sensation at night followed by full blown lesions the next morning, with the face, neck, and arms being the most common sites. Clinically, the most common presentation is linear, erythematous plaques and erythemato-vesicles with a "burnt" appearance and a grey necrotic centre. "Kissing" lesions are common in flexures (Padhi et al., 2007).

The children present with blister beetle dermatitis is not uncommon in tropical climate in regions with paddy and sugarcane. Wearing minimal clothes and sleeping bare-trunked in the hot humid climate predispose to this skin problem. Most of them are unaware of the contact with insects. Repeated incidences are reported in harvesting period when insects are common, and the bizarre shape and recurrent nature may lead to the fear of a "witch spell" in a rural setting.

Investigations

This is a clinical diagnosis.

Management

Antihistamines with mild to moderate topical steroid cure the skin problem.

Preventive measures such as avoiding resting in open areas close to paddy fields and neon lamps during nighttime are advisable.

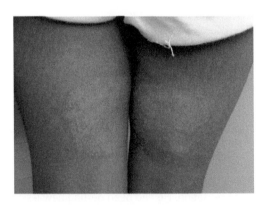

FIGURE 3.4A   A 6-year-old girl came with this itchy, eczematous rash confined to the back of the upper thighs bilaterally. She had recurrences in spite of being treated by her family physician.

Based on the case description and Figure 3.4a, what are your differential diagnoses?

1. Eczema
2. Commode dermatitis or toilet-seat dermatitis
3. Tinea infection

COMMODE DERMATITIS

Diagnosis

Commode dermatitis

Discussion

Commode dermatitis or toilet-seat dermatitis was first described in 1927. At that time, exposure to wooden toilet seats and the associated varnish, lacquers, and paints were to blame for the skin irritation. But even today although the plastic seat covers are used this is common among young children (3–12 years' age), but it is uncommon in adults and in older children. Harsh chemical cleaners containing ingredients such as didecyldimethylammonium chloride and alkyldimethylbenzylammonium chloride, which have previously been documented to cause severe skin irritation, were found to be causative factors (Litvinov et al., 2010; Holme et al., 2005).

Toilet-seat dermatitis causes skin irritation around the buttocks and upper thighs. If it isn't treated properly, discomfort can persist and lead to itchy, painful eczematous rash.

Investigations

This is a clinical diagnosis. Bilateral symmetrical involvement in buttocks and upper thighs is a clue to diagnosis. Some may have a clear imprint of the toilet seat cover on the skin.

Management

Mild to moderate topical steroid with antihistamines would cure the problem, but, advice on prevention is very important.

To prevent recurrences:

- Use toilet seat covers in public restrooms, including hospital and school bathrooms.
- Replace wooden toilet seats with plastic ones.
- Avoid harsh cleaners.

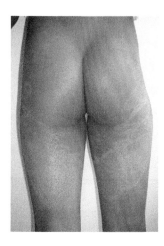

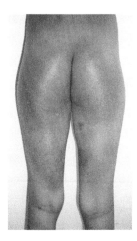

FIGURE 3.4B Commode dermatitis in a 10-year-old boy. Note the clear and complete imprint of the toilet seat cover on the buttocks and upper thighs.

FIGURE 3.4C Commode dermatitis and post-inflammatory hyperpigmentation in an 8-year-old boy.

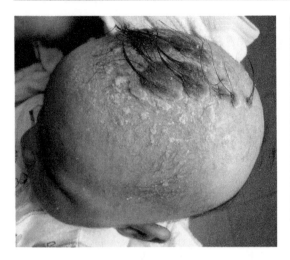

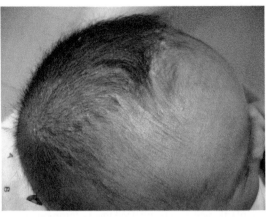

FIGURE 3.5B   A mild cradle cap confined to the scalp is very common.

FIGURE 3.5A   A 3-month-old baby girl was brought with itchy scaly rash on the scalp. She had erythema and scaling in upper torso and other flexures such as bilateral axillae, neck creases, and arm and leg creases.

Based on the case description and Figure 3.5a, what are your differential diagnoses?

1. Cradle cap
2. Infantile seborrhoeic dermatitis
3. Langerhans cell histiocytosis

CRADLE CAP

Diagnosis

Cradle cap

Discussion

Cradle cap can occur in isolation or in association with seborrhoeic dermatitis. Large flakes of yellowish scales are seen on the scalp, especially over the vertex and frontal regions, and may become matted into large plaques of crust. Mild cases are very common, but the condition can become quite extensive. The condition is asymptomatic and the infant is always well; however the disorder may be a source of parental concern (Victoire, 2019). Erythema can be subtle and mislead the severity assessment in darker-skinned infants.

In extensive cases, Langerhans cell histiocytosis (LCH) should be considered, but in LCH the lesional skin tends to ooze, and systemic features may be apparent. Unusual persistence of "cradle cap" or "nappy rash" even in infancy should suggest the possibility of LCH and warrants a biopsy (Higgins & Glover, 2016).

Investigations

This is a clinical diagnosis.

Management

Most cases of cradle cap resolve spontaneously after a few weeks. An emollient will help to lift the scales, and should be used in combination with an appropriate antifungal shampoo.

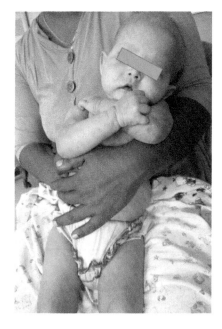

FIGURE 3.6A A 4-month-old baby girl was brought with generalized intractable itching and excoriations. She developed these symptoms one month ago. Note the difference in skin colour between the mother and the baby; father was also close to mother's skin colour.

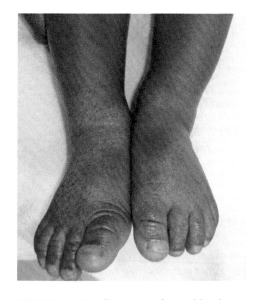

FIGURE 3.6B Extensor dermatitis in a 6-month-old baby (infantile phase: crawling baby).

Based on the case description and Figure 3.6a, what are your differential diagnoses?

1. Infantile seborrhoeic dermatitis
2. Atopic dermatitis/atopic eczema
3. Langerhans cell histiocytosis (LCH)

ECZEMA

Diagnosis

Atopic eczema (AE)

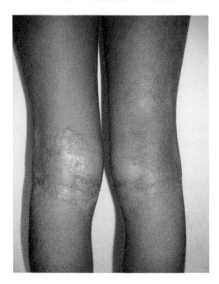

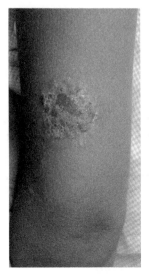

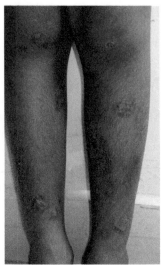

FIGURE 3.6C Flexural dermatitis in a 6-year-old child (childhood phase).

FIGURE 3.6D AND 3.6E Discoid eczema in a 4-year-old girl (childhood phase).

Discussion

Atopic eczema (AE) is an itchy, chronic or chronically relapsing inflammatory skin condition that often starts in early childhood, usually before 2 years of age (Hanifin & Rajka, 1980, De et al., 2006). The rash is characterized by erythema, itchy papules/papulovesicles which may become excoriated and lichenified, and typically has a flexural distribution (Ranawaka, 2021b). The papules are intensely itchy, and may become exudative and crusted as a result of rubbing. Secondary infection and lymphadenopathy are common. In the majority of infants AE clears over time: 43.2% of children with early AE are in complete remission by age 3 years (Ingram, 2016).

The pattern of the rash varies with age (Ardern-Jones et al., 2016):

Infantile phase: The lesions most frequently start on the face, commonly on the cheeks, but may occur anywhere on the skin surface. They subsequently spread to involve the chest and limbs depending on the severity; often the napkin area is relatively spared. When the child begins to crawl, the exposed surfaces, especially the extensor aspect of the knees and elbows, are most involved.

Childhood phase: From 18 to 24 months onwards, the sites most characteristically involved are the elbow and knee

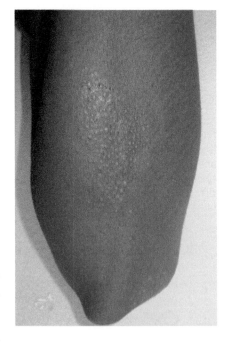

FIGURE 3.6F Follicular accentuation in atopic eczema (childhood phase).

flexures. In some children, a more nummular (discoid) pattern occurs, particularly on the back and legs, which may be mistaken for tinea corporis.

Adult phase: The picture is essentially similar to that in later childhood, with lichenification, especially of the flexures and hands.

Investigations

This is a clinical diagnosis. Skin biopsy was performed in this child to exclude Langerhans cell histiocytosis since the child was having intractable itching in spite of conventional treatments for AE prescribed by her family physician.

Management

The management of infantile atopic eczema for the most part is topical, and primarily aimed at restoring skin barrier function, reducing inflammation, treating secondary infection, and providing parental education and support.

Even though there was no clear-cut evidence of scabies, firstly, this child was treated with 2% permethrin lotion for 24 hours. Then, she was treated with antihistamines, topical diluted betamethasone twice daily, and moisturizers (aqueous cream) applied several times in between, to which she responded remarkably. Her skin colour returned to parental skin colour within 3 months of complete clearance of her AE.

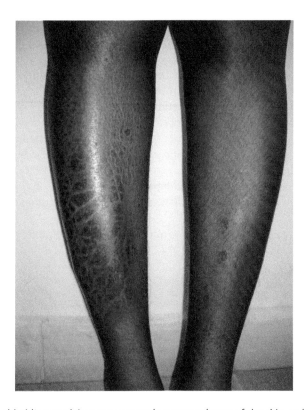

FIGURE 3.7   A 12-year-old girl's complaint was a recently appeared area of dry skin on her right leg. Examination did not reveal similar skin changes anywhere else in the body. This was an acquired ichthyosis on her right leg.

Based on the case description and Figure 3.7, what are your differential diagnoses for acquired ichthyosis in this child?

1. Leprosy present as acquired ichthyosis
2. Drug induced—clofazimine, diuretics (but unlikely to be localized)
3. Cutaneous T-cell lymphoma
4. Cutaneous sarcoidosis/ichthyosiform sarcoidosis (very rare in Asian skin)

ICHTHYOSIS—ACQUIRED

Diagnosis

Acquired ichthyosis or ichthyosis acquisita

Discussion

Acquired ichthyosis is a condition that arises in adulthood but is clinically and histopathologically similar to hereditary ichthyosis vulgaris. It is not, however, inherited but is associated with a systemic disorder.

Disorders which have been associated with acquired ichthyosis are (Chu & Teixeira, 2016):

- *Neoplasia:* particularly Hodgkin disease, mycosis fungoides, multiple myeloma, Kaposi and other sarcomas, and carcinomas (lung, breast, ovary, cervix)
- *Medications:* statins, nicotinic acid, cimetidine, clofazimine
- *Endocrinopathies:* diabetes, thyroid disease, hyperparathyroidism and hypopituitarism
- *Infections:* leprosy, tuberculosis, HIV disease, and HTLV-1 associated myelopathy
- *Autoimmune conditions:* dermatomyositis, systemic lupus erythematosus, and scleroderma/lupus overlap syndrome
- *Chronic metabolic derangements:* including malnutrition, malabsorption syndromes, essential fatty acid deficiency, and pancreatic insufficiency (Shwachman syndrome)
- *Anorexia nervosa*
- *Miscellaneous:* sarcoidosis, bone marrow transplantation, and chronic renal failure

Investigations

The diagnosis of acquired ichthyosis is made clinically. Appropriate investigations should be performed to identify potential causes. In this patient the skin biopsy was performed from the lesion and histopathology confirmed leprosy.

Management

Treat the causative factor. Bland emollients (e.g., emulsifying ointment, Vaseline, or aqueous cream), or 10–12% urea containing moisturizers to the dry skin are recommended.

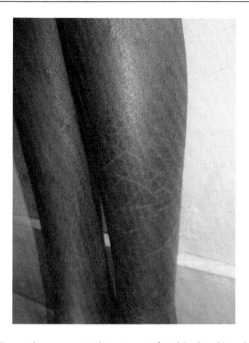

FIGURE 3.8   A 7-year-old girl's mother requested treatment for this dry skin which she had had since infancy.

Based on the case description and Figure 3.8, what are your differential diagnoses?

1. Ichthyosis vulgaris (IV) or autosomal dominant ichthyosis
2. Dry skin

ICHTHYOSIS VULGARIS OR AUTOSOMAL DOMINANT ICHTHYOSIS

Diagnosis

Ichthyosis vulgaris

Discussion

This is an autosomal dominant ichthyosis vulgaris that is a very common skin problem. Filaggrin mutations resulted in impaired epidermal barrier formation and a marked reduction of natural moisturizing factors which play a critical role in hydration of the stratum corneum (Oji et al., 2016). Filaggrin mutations also predispose to atopic eczema (AE), allergic rhinitis, asthma, food allergies, hand eczema, nickel sensitization, and eczema herpeticatum in AE. Therefore, these conditions co-exist in most patients with ichthyosis vulgaris. Ichthyosis vulgaris patients present with light grey scales covering mainly the extensor surfaces of the extremities and the trunk. The scales tend to be smaller, and the groin and larger flexures are always spared. Almost all ichthyosis vulgaris patients show accentuated palmar creases (Jaffar, 2022).

Investigations

This is a clinical diagnosis.

Management

Ointments that hydrate the stratum corneum are beneficial: creams containing glycerol, urea-containing creams (up to 10%), or creams containing lactic acid up to 12% work well. Excessive bathing procedures are not necessary, but showering and subsequent application of ointments is advisable.

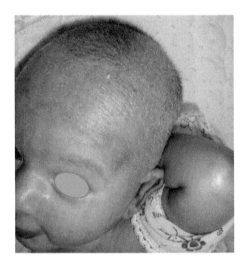

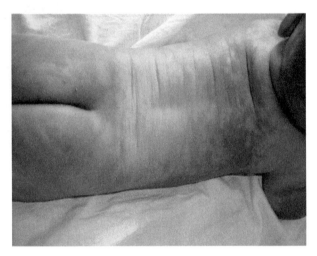

FIGURE 3.9A A 3-month-old baby was brought with itchy, erythematous scalp and flexures.

FIGURE 3.9B Infantile seborrhoeic dermatitis in a 2-month-old baby showing post-inflammatory hypopigmentation at the back of the trunk.

Based on the case description and Figure 3.9a, what are your differential diagnoses?

1. Infantile seborrhoeic dermatitis
2. Atopic dermatitis

INFANTILE SEBORRHOEIC DERMATITIS/CRADLE CAP

Diagnosis

Infantile seborrhoeic dermatitis (ISD)

Discussion

Typically, ISD occurs between the ages of 4 and 12 weeks, but most commonly before the age of 2 months (64%) with 28% occurring later, between 2 and 4 months (Higgins & Glover, 2016). ISD is mostly asymptomatic, but may cause great parental concern. Mostly the erythema occurs in the skin folds, especially the neck and the inguinal regions, but may be severe to involve the scalp and eyebrows characteristically with erythema and scales, and may be associated with cradle cap. Typically, the inflammation resolves with transient hypopigmentation, which is pronounced in children with darker skin colour.

Investigations

This is a clinical diagnosis.

Management

In mild cases, treatment with emollient alone is effective. Steroid–antifungal combination creams are often employed in cases in which inflammation is marked, but should only be used sparsely, and for a short period.

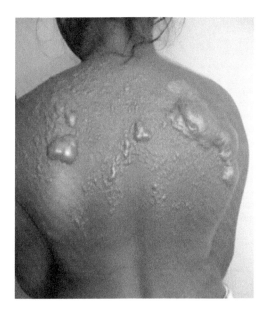

FIGURE 3.10   A 9-year-old girl came with this acute blistering eruption within a few hours after applying 5% permethrin.

Based on the case description and Figure 3.10, what are your differential diagnoses?

1. Irritant contact dermatitis to permethrin
2. Blistering disease

IRRITANT CONTACT DERMATITIS

Diagnosis

Irritant contact dermatitis

Discussion

Irritant contact dermatitis is the cutaneous response to the physical/toxic effects of a wide range of environmental exposures. This may be an acute (toxic) irritant contact dermatitis or a cumulative irritant/insult dermatitis. Irritant contact dermatitis has a spectrum of clinical features, ranging from a little dryness, redness, or chapping through various types of eczematous dermatitis to an acute caustic burn. The same chemical may cause different irritant reactions depending on the concentration and the individual response (White, 2016).

Investigations

This is a clinical diagnosis.

Management

Symptomatic treatment and educate on the causative factor.

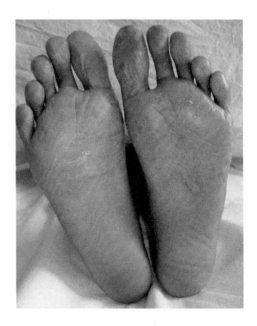

FIGURE 3.11   A 10-year-old girl complained of soreness of soles, mainly forefoot.

Based on the case description and Figure 3.11, what are your differential diagnoses?

1. Juvenile plantar dermatosis or forefoot eczema
2. Tinea pedis
3. Footwear allergy

JUVENILE PLANTAR DERMATOSIS

Diagnosis

Juvenile plantar dermatosis or forefoot eczema

Discussion

The presenting features of juvenile plantar dermatosis are redness and soreness on the plantar surface of the forefoot. On examination, shiny, dry, fissured dermatitis of the plantar surface of the forefoot is noted. It occurs mainly in children aged 3–14 years, but occasionally in adults or infants. The symmetry of the lesions is a striking feature. The toe clefts are normal and this helps to distinguish the condition from tinea pedis. Most cases will clear spontaneously during childhood or adolescence (Silverberg, 2017; Ahn et al., 2017).

Investigations

This is a clinical diagnosis. Skin scrapings to exclude fungus and patch tests to exclude footwear allergy may be helpful in doubtful cases.

Management

Change footwear to cotton socks and open sandals. Frequent application of emollients, including urea-containing preparations is recommended. Topical tacrolimus ointment (Protopic TM) may help in resistant cases.

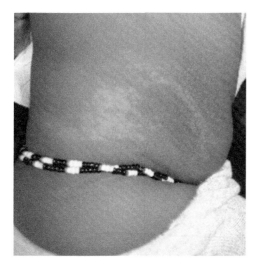

FIGURE 3.12A   A 7-month-old girl came with an asymptomatic, skin-coloured linear lesion that appeared two weeks ago, and extended rapidly along her right flank.

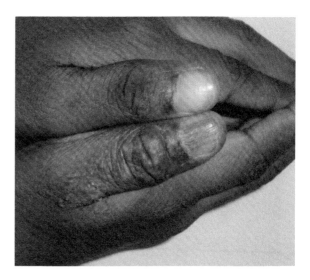

FIGURE 3.12B   Lichen striatus along the right thumb extending to the nail (nail lichen striatus).

Based on the case description and Figure 3.12a, what are your differential diagnoses?

1. Lichen striatus
2. Linear epidermal naevus
3. Linear lichen planus

LICHEN STRIATUS

Diagnosis

Lichen striatus

Discussion

Lichen striatus is a self-limiting and asymptomatic inflammatory dermatosis characterized by hypopigmented or skin-coloured linear distribution that develops in the lines of Blaschko. It's common in children aged 5 to 15 years, but may appear in infants and adults, too (Piguet et al., 2016). The initial presentation is characterized by the sudden appearance of small, discrete, skin-coloured, flat-topped, lichenoid papules in a typical linear distribution. The lesions occur most commonly (over 75%) on one arm or leg, or on the neck, but may develop on the trunk. Involvement of the nails may result in longitudinal ridging, splitting, onycholysis, or nail loss (Leung et al., 2020).

The onset is usually sudden, typically reaches its maximum extent within 2–3 weeks, and generally resolves over 6–12 months, but may persist for several years.

Investigations

This is a clinical diagnosis.

Management

Observation and reassurance. Topical corticosteroids if itchy. Topical corticosteroids, topical tacrolimus, or topical pimecrolimus may help in resistant cases.

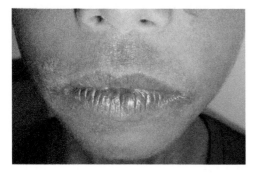

FIGURE 3.13A A 7-year-old boy came with itchy, eczematous lesions around his mouth. Even though it responds to the treatments prescribed by his family doctor, it has been recurring for the last 3 months. Note the dry fissured lips.

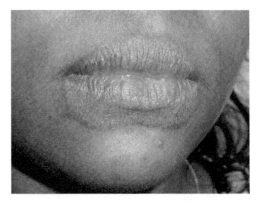

FIGURE 3.13B Post-inflammatory hyperpigmentation following lip lick dermatitis. Note the dry, eczematous lips which is the initiating factor.

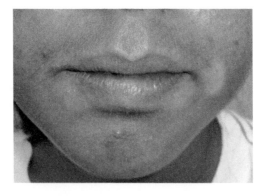

FIGURE 3.13C Post-inflammatory hypopigmentation following lip lick dermatitis.

Based on the case description and Figure 3.13a, what are your differential diagnoses?

1. Lip lick dermatitis or lip-lick chelitis
2. Perioral dermatitis

LIP LICK DERMATITIS

Diagnosis

Lip lick dermatitis/lip lick cheilitis

Discussion

Dry, cracked lips are a common occurrence in both cold months and arid climates, leading many patients to experience discomfort. Lip-licking is a compensatory measure that perpetuates the condition and often leads to lip-licking dermatitis in patients in whom this compensatory measure becomes a chronic habit. Lip lick dermatitis is a moist or fissured eczema (Silverberg, 2017) around the mouth that is common in children and even adults. It frequently spreads to some distance around the mouth, and is associated with dry lips and cheilitis. It may become eczematous or leave post-inflammatory hyperpigmentation or hypopigmentation. Its origin is mostly related to habits of lip-licking, thumb-sucking, dribbling, or chapping (Fonseca et al., 2020).

In perioral dermatitis, the papules and pustules present on an erythematous and/or scaling base, localized symmetrically around the mouth with a clear zone around the vermillion border. This eruption is implicated to the use of topical corticosteroids on the face or inhaled corticosteroid use. Perioral dermatitis is not common in our setting since steroids are rarely used on the face.

Investigations

This is a clinical diagnosis. While taking the history observe the child (or the adult) for the habit of lip-licking since they do it involuntarily and often deny it.

Management

Mild steroid with emollient to the eczematous area would cure the problem.

Educate the parents and the child on the causative factors and advise to get rid of the habit. If dry lips are the causative factor, frequent moisturizer to the lips is important until the habit of lip-licking stops.

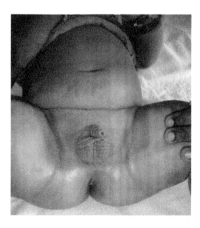

FIGURE 3.14A A 3-month-old baby was brought with this erythematous rash on perineal area. Note the erythema extends to lower abdomen and buttocks, and skin folds are spared.

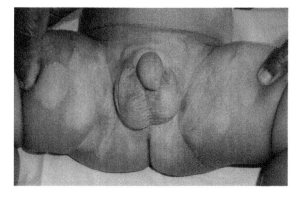

FIGURE 3.14B Note the erythema and hypopigmentation is confined to the nappy area, which favours the diagnosis of nappy rash.

Based on the case description and Figure 3.14a, what are your differential diagnoses?

1. Irritant napkin dermatitis/nappy rash/napkin (diaper) dermatitis
2. Infantile seborrhoeic dermatitis
3. Infantile psoriasis

NAPKIN DERMATITIS

Diagnosis

Nappy rash

Discussion

Prolonged contact with urine induces an irritant erythema which may lead to erosions if untreated. This is more common where traditional cloth nappies are still in use. Involved areas are those in contact with the irritant (e.g., the buttocks, front and back of the lower trunk). The skin folds may be spared in contrast to seborrhoeic dermatitis or infantile psoriasis (Fölster-Holst, 2018). Persistent diaper dermatitis not responding to conventional treatments should arouse the suspicion of Langerhans cell histiocytosis in infants (Moscona-Nissan, 2022).

Post-inflammatory hypopigmentation which last for many months even after the rash is cured is common in dark-skinned babies.

Investigations

This is a clinical diagnosis.

Management

Treatment is aimed at keeping the skin dry and using barrier creams or emollients to restore normal epidermis. Topical steroids should only be used in the short term, and only if inflammation is severe.

Secondary infection should be treated appropriately (Hebert, 2021).

Advise to parents to use modern disposable nappies (diapers) during the night, which are much more absorbent, to prevent recurrences. Wearing diapers during the daytime may be uncomfortable in the hot humid climate of the tropics.

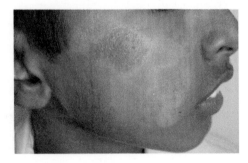

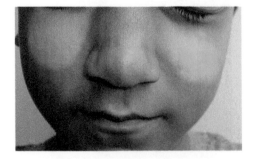

FIGURE 3.15A A 9-year-old boy came with itchy eczematous rash on the face bilaterally for 3 months. This started as mildly itchy hypopigmented patches on the face, that progressed to eczematous rash after few months.

FIGURE 3.15B PLE starting as an asymptomatic well-demarcated hypopigmented patches on the highest sun-exposed sites are common in darker-skinned children. In many of them this is the only skin manifestation of PLE.

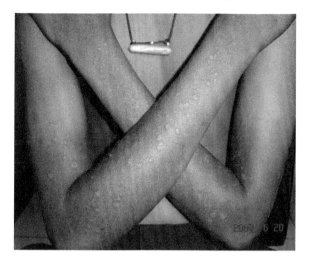

FIGURE 3.15C   PLE appears as discrete papular and eczematous eruption in a 10-year-old boy. Note the extensor involvement and sharp cut-off at sites of photoprotection at the shirt arm line.

Based on the case description and Figure 3.15a, what are your differential diagnoses?

1. Photodermatitis/polymorphic light eruption (PLE)
2. Atopic eczema
3. Pityriasis versicolor

PHOTODERMATITIS

Diagnosis

Polymorphic light eruption

Discussion

Polymorphic light eruption (PLE) is a recurrent, delayed-onset, abnormal reaction to sunlight (or artificial UVR source) that resolves without scarring. There are several morphological variants, hence the term "polymorphic" (Ibbotson & Dawe, 2016). Exposure to ultraviolet radiation and occasionally visible light and artificial lights (that is used inside buildings) are important in the manifestation of PLE. Polymorphic light eruption affects sunlight-exposed sites exclusively, such as the cheeks, dorsal forearms, dorsal hands, and dorsal feet. Even this can extend to the trunk when children play outdoors bare-trunked as is common in the tropics. It is mostly seen in older children who are allowed to play outdoors. In extensive sunburn or PLE, a lack of involvement and sharp cut-off at sites of photoprotection may be seen (de Silva, 2021). The upper eyelids, creases under the eyes, shaded areas under the lower lip and chin, and behind the ears, which are usually sun-protected, are notably spared.

Investigations

This is a clinical diagnosis.

Management

Management involves photoprotection and mild steroids if itchy. Post-inflammatory hypopigmentation may last for months and reassurance and education may relieve parental anxiety.

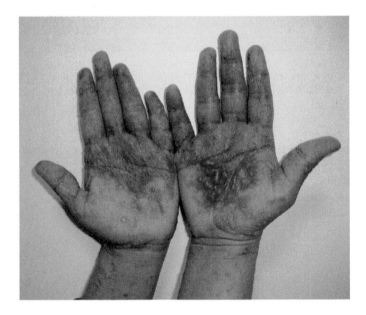

FIGURE 3.16   This 12-year-old Muslim girl had decorated her palms using henna (Mindi), and after 24 hours she had developed these itchy, eczematous, vesicular-bullous eruption on palms and dorsum of hands.

Based on the case description and Figure 3.16, what are your differential diagnoses?

1. Phytophotodermatitis
2. Irritant contact dermatitis

PHYTOPHOTODERMATITIS

Diagnosis

Phytophotodermatitis

Discussion

Phytophotodermatitis is an inflammatory and pigmentary reaction of the skin to light, potentiated by furocoumarins in plants (Sheehan, 2020). The reaction occurs in those exposed to sunlight after skin contact with these plants, especially if they have been crushed. Intensely pruritic papulovesicular lesions with irregular shapes and criss-crossing linear streaks may be present or multiple irregular large bullae may form.

Depending on the site and the type of plant contact this may mimic irritant contact dermatitis or blister beetle dermatitis.

Investigations

This is a clinical diagnosis.

Management

Symptomatic management with oral antihistamines, topical or oral antibiotics, and/or topical or systemic steroids, depending on the severity. Parenterally administered epinephrine in case of anaphylactic reactions is recommended. Avoidance of photodynamic or phototoxic drugs, plants and perfumes are important to prevent recurrences.

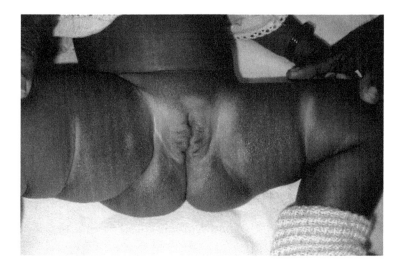

FIGURE 3.17   A 7-month-old baby was brought with asymptomatic hypopigmented patches on flexures and the trunk for one month's duration.

Based on the case description and Figure 3.17, what are your differential diagnoses?

1. Post-inflammatory hypopigmentation
2. Vitiligo

POST-INFLAMMATORY HYPOPIGMENTATION

Diagnosis

Post-inflammatory hypopigmentation

Discussion

The post-inflammatory hypopigmentation is easily visible and very common in dark-skinned babies. This can occur as a consequence of several diseases: infantile seborrhoeic dermatitis, nappy rash, drooping saliva (around the mouth and neck), drug rash, or atopic eczema. Mostly, they are asymptomatic, but may be itchy if the primary skin problem is an itchy condition, such as an infantile seborrhoeic dermatitis or an atopic eczema (Rao et al., 2023).

Investigations

This is a clinical diagnosis.

Management

Identify the primary cause and treat it. This is a great parental concern that the baby is getting vitiligo; however, reassurance would relieve their tension. Application of mild moisturizers twice daily is sufficient if asymptomatic. This post-inflammatory hypopigmentation may last for months even after the primary course is cured.

REFERENCES

Ahn C, Huang W (2017). Clinical presentation of atopic dermatitis. *Advances in Experimental Medicine and Biology* 1027:39–46. doi: 10.1007/978-3-319-64804-0_4.

Ardern-Jones MR, Flohr C, Reynolds NJ, Holden CA (2016). Atopic eczema. In Christopher G, Jonathan B, Tanya B, Robert C, Daniel C, eds. *Rook's Textbook of Dermatology*, 9th edn. Hoboken: Wiley-Blackwell, 41.20p.

Chu AC, Teixeira F (2016). Acquired disorders of epidermal keratinization. In Christopher G, Jonathan B, Tanya B, Robert C, Daniel C, eds. Rook's Textbook of Dermatology, 9th edn. Hoboken: Wiley-Blackwell, 87.1p.

De D, Kanwar AJ, Handa S (2006). Comparative efficacy of Hanifin and Rajka's criteria and the UK working party's diagnostic criteria in diagnosis of atopic dermatitis in a hospital setting in North India. *Journal of the European Academy of Dermatology and Venereology*;20(7):853–9. doi: 10.1111/j.1468-3083.2006.01664.x.

de Silva H (2021). Photodermatosis. In Ranawaka RR, Kannangara AP, Karawita, A, eds. *Atlas of Dermatoses in Pigmented Skin*. Singapore: Springer, pp. 183–200. doi: 10.1007/978-981-15-5483-4_10.

Fölster-Holst R (2018). Differential diagnoses of diaper dermatitis. *Pediatric Dermatology*;35(Suppl 1):s10–8. doi: 10.1111/pde.13484.

Fonseca A, Jacob SE, Sindle A (2020). Art of prevention: Practical interventions in lip-licking dermatitis. *International Journal of Women's Dermatology* 5;6(5):377–80. doi: 10.1016/j.ijwd.2020. 06.001.

Hanifin and Rajka (1980). Diagnostic criteria of atopic dermatitis/eczema. *Acta Dermatology and Venereology* (Stockh) 1980;(Suppl 92):44–7.

Hebert AA (2021). A new therapeutic horizon in diaper dermatitis: Novel agents with novel action. *International Journal of Women's Dermatology* 16;7(4):466–70. doi: 10.1016/j.ijwd.2021.02.003.

Higgins EM, Glover MT. (2016) Dermatoses and haemangiomas of infancy. In Christopher G, Jonathan B, Tanya B, Robert C, Daniel C, eds. *Rook's Textbook of Dermatology*, 9th edn. Hoboken: Wiley-Blackwell, 117.3p.

Holme SA, Stone NM, Mills CM. (2005) Toilet seat contact dermatitis. *Pediatric Dermatology*;22(4):344–5. doi: 10.1111/j.1525-1470.2005.22413.x.

Ibbotson S, Dawe R (2016). Cutaneous photosensitivity diseases. In Christopher G, Jonathan B, Tanya B, Robert C, Daniel C, eds. *Rook's Textbook of Dermatology*, 9th edn. Hoboken: Wiley-Blackwell, 127.2p.

Ingram JR (2016). Eczematous disorders. In Christopher G, Jonathan B, Tanya B, Robert C, Daniel C, eds. *Rook's Textbook of Dermatology*, 9th edn. Hoboken: Wiley-Blackwell, 39.1p.

Jaffar H, Shakir Z, Kumar G, Ali IF (2022). Ichthyosis vulgaris: An updated review. *Skin Health & Disease* 25;3(1):e187. doi: 10.1002/ski2.187.

Leung AKC, Leong KF, Barankin B (2020). Lichen striatus with nail involvement in a 6-Year-old boy. *Case Reports in Pediatrics* 27;2020:1494760. doi: 10.1155/2020/1494760.

Litvinov IV, Sugathan P, Cohen BA (2010). Recognizing and treating toilet-seat contact dermatitis in children. *Pediatrics*;125(2):e419–22. doi: 10.1542/peds.2009-2430.

Moscona-Nissan A, Maldonado-Colin G, Romo-López A, Ventura-Zarate A (2022). Langerhans cell histiocytosis presented as persistent diaper dermatitis: A case report. *Cureus* 6;14(7):e26606. doi: 10.7759/cureus.26606.

Oji V, Dieter Metze D, Traupe H (2016). Inherited disorders of cornification. In Christopher G, Jonathan B, Tanya B, Robert C, Daniel C, eds. *Rook's Textbook of Dermatology*, 9th edn. Hoboken: Wiley-Blackwell, 65.1p.

Padhi T, Mohanty P, Jena S, Sirka CS, Mishra S (2007). Clinicoepidemiological profile of 590 cases of beetle dermatitis in western Orissa. *The Indian Journal of Dermatology, Venereology and Leprology* 73:333–5.

Piguet V, Breathnach SM, Cleach LL (2016) Lichen planus and lichenoid disorders. In Christopher G, Jonathan B, Tanya B, Robert C, Daniel C, eds. *Rook's Textbook of Dermatology*, 9th edn. Hoboken: Wiley-Blackwell, 37.18p.

Ranawaka RR (2021a). Allergic and irritant contact dermatitis. In Ranawaka RR, Kannangara AP, Karawita A, eds. *Atlas of Dermatoses in Pigmented Skin*. Singapore: Springer, pp. 151–68. doi: 10.1007/978-981-15-5483-4_8

Ranawaka RR (2021b). Eczematous disorders. In Ranawaka RR, Kannangara AP, Karawita A, eds. *Atlas of Dermatoses in Pigmented Skin*. Singapore: Springer, pp. 107–22. doi: 10.1007/978-981-15-5483-4_6

Rao M, Young K, Jackson-Cowan L, Kourosh A, Theodosakis N (2023). Post-inflammatory hypopigmentation: Review of the etiology, clinical manifestations, and treatment options. *Journal of Clinical Medicine* 3;12(3):1243. doi: 10.3390/jcm12031243.

Sheehan MP (2020). Plant associated irritant & allergic contact dermatitis (phytodermatitis). *Dermatologic Clinics*;38(3):389–98. doi: 10.1016/j.det.2020.02.010.

Silverberg NB (2017). Typical and atypical clinical appearance of atopic dermatitis. *Clinics in Dermatology*;35(4):354–9. doi: 10.1016/j.clindermatol.2017.03.007.

Srihari S, Kombettu AP, Rudrappa KG, Betkerur J (2017). Paederus dermatitis: A case series. *Indian Dermatology Online Journal*;8(5):361–4.

Srisaravanapavananthan, F. (2021). Cultural dermatoses. In Ranawaka RR, Kannangara AP, Karawita A, eds. *Atlas of Dermatoses in Pigmented Skin*. Singapore: Springer, pp. 797–802. doi: 10.1007/978-981-15-5483-4_39.

van Geel N, Speeckaert R (2016). Acquired pigmentary disorders. In Christopher G, Jonathan B, Tanya B, Robert C, Daniel C, eds. *Rook's Textbook of Dermatology*, 9th edn. Hoboken: Wiley-Blackwell, 88.28p.

Victoire A, Magin P, Coughlan J, van Driel ML (2019). Interventions for infantile seborrhoeic dermatitis (including cradle cap). *Cochrane Database of Systematic Reviews* 4;3(3):CD011380. doi: 10.1002/14651858. CD011380.pub2.

White JML (2016) Irritant contact dermatitis. In Christopher G, Jonathan B, Tanya B, Robert C, Daniel C, eds. *Rook's Textbook of Dermatology*, 9th edn. Hoboken: Wiley-Blackwell, 129.1p.

Common Dermatoses in Children with FST 5

4

Ranthilaka R. Gammanpila

INTRODUCTION

This chapter discusses 12 common dermatological problems we encounter in children with brown skin (Fitzpatrick skin type V/FST 5) using 16 clinical photographs. These are discussed based on a clinical photograph and easy-to-read question-and-answer format. Erythema is inconspicuous and post-inflammatory hypopigmentation and hyperpigmentation are marked in coloured-skinned children. For example, PASI score in psoriasis is much lower in a darker-skinned child of the same severity due to 0 or 1 erythema score; genital lichen sclerosus presents early as darker-skinned children notice depigmentation, mistaken for vitiligo, and seek early medical attention. Early initiation of treatment results in good prognosis in lichen sclerosus and morphoea in darker-skinned patients.

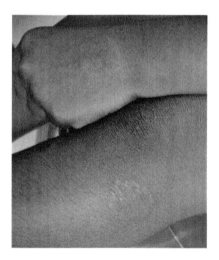

FIGURE 4.1   A 9-year-old girl came with these asymptomatic lesions on her limbs for one month's duration.

Based on the case description and Figure 4.1, what are your differential diagnoses?

1. Granuloma annulare
2. Tinea infection
3. Morphoea

GRANULOMA ANNULARE

Diagnosis

Granuloma annulare (localized)

Discussion

The typical presentation is of annular indurated papules and/or plaques on the extremities, which slowly enlarge. They eventually flatten and fade over months or years. Granuloma annulare is most common in children and young adults but can occur at any age, and is more common in women. Most are asymptomatic, but may be tender or itchy.

Several different clinical types are seen: localized, generalized, subcutaneous, and perforating (Joshi & Duvic, 2022).

- *Localized GA* accounts for about three quarters of cases and typically presents as a ring of small, smooth, skin-coloured papules or plaques. Stretching the skin enables the papules or plaques to be seen more readily. They may be solitary or multiple, and may occur anywhere on the skin, although the dorsa of the hands, knuckles, fingers, and feet are the commonest sites (Figure 4.1).
- *Generalized GA* occurs more commonly in adults with a mean around 50 years. This is the commonest form seen in HIV patients.
- *Subcutaneous GA* is uncommon. It occurs predominantly in children. Subcutaneous GA is clinically and histologically similar to a rheumatoid nodule with large areas of necrobiosis.
- *Perforating GA* has been reported in both adults and children. Localized or generalized papules develop yellowish centres and discharge a little clear, viscous fluid that dries to form a crust, eventually separating to leave a hypo- or hyperpigmented scar.

Investigations

This is a clinical diagnosis, confirmed with histopathology. The most characteristic histological lesion in GA is the necrobiotic granuloma.

Management

In most cases, particularly in children, reassurance of eventual resolution is all that is needed. For generalized disease, PUVA appears to give the best results (Wang & Khachemoune, 2018).

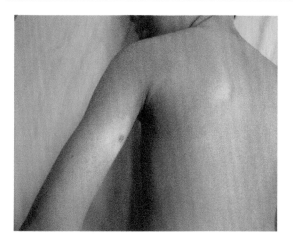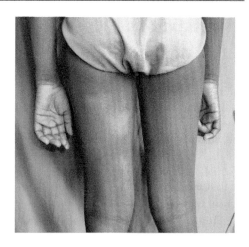

FIGURE 4.2A, 4.2B   An 8-year-old boy presented with hypopigmented patches on the limbs and trunk. He was otherwise asymptomatic and sensation was normal over the lesions.

Based on the case description and Figure 4.2a and b, what are your differential diagnoses?

1. Leprosy
2. Pityriasis versicolor
3. Hypopigmented mycosis fungoides
4. Vitiligo

HYPOPIGMENTED MYCOSIS FUNGOIDES

Diagnosis

Hypopigmented mycosis fungoides (HMF)

Discussion

The most common type of primary cutaneous T-cell lymphoma (CTCL) is mycosis fungoides. In dark-skinned patients hypopigmented MF is the commonest clinical variant that is asymptomatic and confined to non-sun-exposed areas. HMF has predilection for dark-skinned individuals of African, West Indian, or Asian origin. The incidence of HMF in white Caucasians is rare with few cases reported. Patients with HMF are younger (mean of 29 years) than classical MF (mean of 63 years). Overall survival rate and disease-specific survival rates at 5 and 10 years were 100% in hypopigmented MF and stage 1A disease, and disease progression at 5 and 10 years was 0% in HMF in a study published by Wain et al. (Wain, 2003). In a tropical climate, exposure to natural sunlight possibly cures the lesions on sun-exposed areas at early stage of onset. HMF resembles clinically very common hypopigmented skin conditions leading to a mean of 36 months of diagnostic delay (Ranawaka et al., 2011; Ranawaka, 2021a).

Investigations

Selecting the biopsy site is very important in these cases; the most depigmented patch on covered body area with least interference with treatments should be selected, e.g., buttocks, back of the trunk. Usually two or more biopsies are performed from different sites. It is well known that the clinical diagnosis proceeds histological confirmation by many years.

Histologically, HMF lesions tend to show marked epidermotropism, in contrast to the subtle clinical features, and loss of melanocytes probably due to a direct cytotoxic effect of the CD8+ tumour cells.

The pathological diagnosis of early MF can be extremely subjective and clinicopathological correlation is essential. Sequential biopsies at 3–6-month intervals may be needed in doubtful cases since the clinical picture evolves over a period of months or even years.

Management

Since the HMF runs an indolent course, aggressive treatment is not recommended in children. The authors have found following therapies are effective in children with HMF:

1. Topical potent steroids
2. Topical 0.1% tacrolimus
3. Combination of topical steroids and tacrolimus alternatively
4. The foregoing may be combined with natural sunlight exposure 20 minutes per day, 3–4 days per week.

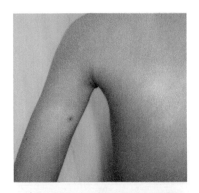

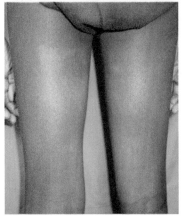

FIGURE 4.2C, 4.2D   This child was treated with topical steroids and topical 0.1% tacrolimus on alternate days and natural sunlight exposure 20 minutes per session for 3 days per week. After 10 weeks he showed marked clinical improvement.

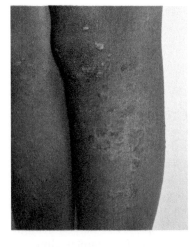

FIGURE 4.3   A 7-year-old girl came with itchy hyperpigmented lesions on her limbs and trunk for 2 months.

Based on the case description and Figure 4.3, what are your differential diagnoses?

1. Cutaneous lichen planus
2. Post-inflammatory hyperpigmentation

LICHEN PLANS (LP)

Diagnosis

Lichen planus (cutaneous and widespread)

Discussion

The classic clinical presentation of lichen planus (LP) includes primary lesions consisting of firm, shiny, polygonal, 1–3-mm diameter papules with a violet to blackish grey colour. Erythematous lesions are uncommon in dark skin (Kannangara, 2021). More closely, a tracery of thin white lines can be seen on the surface of the lesions, known as Wickham's striae. Wickham's striae are more clearly seen in oral LP lesions. Papules can be isolated or grouped, in a linear or annular distribution. Typically, a greyish black pigmentation can be observed in lesions that have resolved due to deposition of melanin in the superficial dermis. LP can affect any part of the body surface, but is most often seen on the volar aspect of the wrists, the lumbar region, and around the ankles.

Pruritus is a fairly consistent feature in LP and ranges from occasional mild irritation to more or less continuous severe itching, which interferes with sleep and makes life almost intolerable; occasionally, pruritus is completely absent.

Investigations

This is a clinical diagnosis. Histopathology would help in doubtful cases. The characteristic histological changes are best seen in biopsies of fully developed LP papules. Colloid bodies, "sawtooth" appearance in rete ridges, band-like infiltrate of lymphocytes and histiocytes, and pigmentary incontinence with dermal melanophages are characteristic (Piguet et al., 2016).

Management

Treatment of LP depends on the localization, clinical form, and severity. For cutaneous LP, which can clear spontaneously within 1–2 years, the aim of treatment is to reduce pruritus and time to resolution. The main therapy for LP is corticosteroids: topical or systemic corticosteroids depend on the severity, commonly recommended as first-line treatment (Melin et al., 2022). Topical tacrolimus 0.1% was found to be equally effective and cause fewer side effects especially on the face, neck, genitals, and flexures, but is more expensive (Özkur et al., 2019).

- *Limited cutaneous LP*: potent topical corticosteroids can be used in children for 2–6 weeks, then continue less frequently during maintenance therapy.
- *Widespread cutaneous LP*: prednisolone 0.5–1 mg/kg per day until improvement, then continue with topical steroids during maintenance therapy.

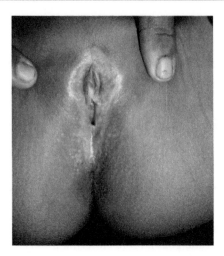

FIGURE 4.4A   A 9-year-old girl came complaining of itchy genitals for two months' duration that did not respond to treatments prescribed by her family doctor. Examination revealed depigmented glazy skin on labia majora.

Based on the case description and Figure 4.4a, what are your differential diagnoses?

1. Vitiligo
2. Lichen sclerosus or lichen sclerosus et atrophicus
3. Sexual abuse
4. Genital candidosis

LICHEN SCLEROSUS

Diagnosis

Lichen sclerosus

Discussion

Lichen sclerosus (LS) is a common inflammatory dermatosis with a predilection for ano-genital skin. This may occur at any age but more common in prepubertal girls and postmenopausal women. Lichen sclerosus is 6–10 times more common in females than in males (Aróstegui Aguilar et al., 2022, Bunker & Porter, 2016).

The presenting symptom is usually itching, which is often severe and distressing. Elderly women may present with discomfort and dyspareunia. Constipation is a common feature in girls with prepubertal disease (Lewis, 2016). LS is characterized by flat, atrophic, whitened epithelium, which may become confluent, extending around the vulval and perianal skin. There may also be oedema, purpura, bullae, erosions, fissures, and ulceration in late disease. Vitiligoid LS is a common presentation

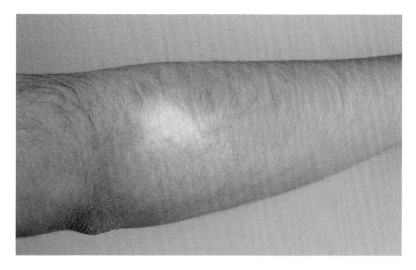

FIGURE 4.4B Extragenital lichen sclerosus in a 16-year-old girl.

in dark-skinned children. Since it is mistaken for vitiligo they present early (Dennin et al., 2018, Veronesi, 2021).

LS may occur extragenitally. The classic lesions seen on the extragenital skin are ivory white papules and plaques (Figure 4.4b). Vitiligo, mucous membrane pemphigoid, lichen planus, and morphoea may present with a similar clinical appearance. Genital LS may be mistaken for sexual abuse; on the contrary, the sexual abuse may be the initiating or exacerbating factor of the LS (Oyama & Hasegawa, 2022). Co-existence of morphoea and lichen sclerosus is well documented (Figure 5.3d).

Investigations

This is a clinical diagnosis in most. Histopathology is performed for confirmation in doubtful cases. The epidermis is atrophic with basal cell hydropic degeneration. The superficial dermis is oedematous and hyalinized. Deep to the hyalinized zone is a band-like lymphohistiocytic infiltrate (Corazza et al., 2021).

Management

- The super-potent topical corticosteroid, clobetasol propionate 0.05%, is the first-line treatment: once nightly for 4 weeks, then alternate nights for 4 weeks, and twice a week for a further month. Vaginal candidosis due to topical steroids is a common side effect in women and children.
- The calcineurin inhibitors tacrolimus or pimecrolimus as steroid-sparing alternatives are preferred in many girls and women due to fewer side effects.
- Surgery is only indicated for the management of functional problems caused by post-inflammatory scarring, premalignant lesions, and malignancy.
- Vitiligoid LS has very good prognosis with complete clearance without sequel because they present early for treatments (Ranawaka, 2021b).

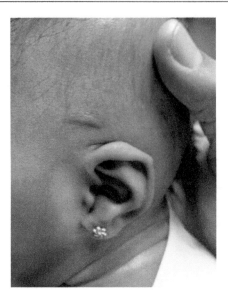

FIGURE 4.5 A 5-month-old baby girl was brought with this mildly itchy papule on her scalp since birth. Her mother had noticed that this lesion becomes enlarged and more prominent after rubbing.

Based on the case description and Figure 4.5, what are your differential diagnoses?

1. Mastocytoma
2. Connective tissue naevus

MASTOCYTOMA

Diagnosis

Mastocytoma

Discussion

Cutaneous mastocytoma may present as skin-coloured nodules or plaques in infancy or early childhood, measuring up to 3–4 cm in diameter. They are usually solitary. Nearly all mastocytomas involute over the first few years of childhood.

Investigations

This is a clinical diagnosis, but can be confirmed histopathologically.

Management

Potent or very potent topical corticosteroids twice daily for 6 weeks are recommended.
    Intralesional injection of corticosteroids into individual mastocytomas gives good results.

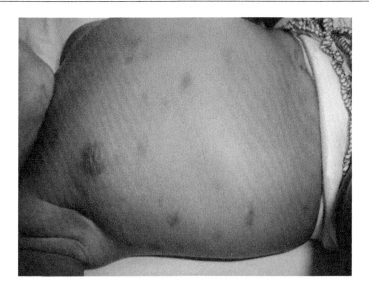

FIGURE 4.6 A 5-month-old baby girl presented with these hyperpigmented patches all over the trunk and limbs for one month. The mother had noticed that these lesions become more prominent and swollen after rubbing the skin during a bath.

Based on the case description and Figure 4.6, what are your differential diagnoses?

1. Post-inflammatory hyperpigmentation
2. Mastocytosis (macular papular type) or urticaria pigmentosa

MASTOCYTOSIS (URTICARIA PIGMENTOSA)

Diagnosis

Mastocytosis (macular papular type or urticaria pigmentosa)

Discussion

Mastocytosis is characterized by too many mast cells in the skin and other tissues. Mastocytosis in infancy is usually limited to the skin, with three distinct clinical presentations: maculopapular (formerly urticaria pigmentosa) (Figure 4.6), diffuse cutaneous mastocytosis, and solitary mastocytoma (Figure 4.5). Clinically, numerous brown macules, maculopapules, plaques, or nodules appear in a symmetrical distribution anywhere on the body except the palms and soles. They characteristically urticate within minutes of gentle rubbing (Darier's sign) in children causing localized pruritus, redness, and wheal, which subside within an hour. Lesions may blister in infancy or childhood and this may be the presenting feature, but they heal without scarring. Flushing, pruritus, heat or cold intolerance, recurrent diarrhoea, acid dyspepsia, urinary frequency, depression, headache, wheezing, or syncope may develop in an acute attack (Tiano, 2022).

Investigations

This is confirmed histopathologically. The epidermis is normal. Mast cell numbers are increased in the dermis. The mast cells are oval- or spindle-shaped with granules that stain metachromatically with toluidine blue. A careful technique when taking the skin biopsy to minimize traumatic degranulation is important. Injecting local anaesthetic around the lesion to be biopsied may yield a higher number of stainable mast cells (Grattan & Radia, 2016).

Management

- Advise on the avoidance of factors known to stimulate mast cell degranulation, such as aspirin, non-steroidal anti-inflammatory drugs, codeine, opiates, polymyxin B, intravenous radiograph contrast fluids, and MRI contrast media. (Sandru et al.,2021)
- Potent or very potent topical corticosteroids twice daily for 6 weeks can lead to clearance of mast cells and reduction of pigmentation.
- Oral corticosteroids at high doses can offer temporary symptomatic improvement for patients with aggressive systemic mastocytosis.
- Symptomatic therapy: H 1 receptor blocker may help control itch, blistering, flushing, and urtication plus an H 2 blocker if there are symptoms of hyperacidity or ulceration with or without oral sodium cromoglycate for diarrhoea.
- Children with a history of anaphylaxis should be supplied with an adrenaline auto injector.

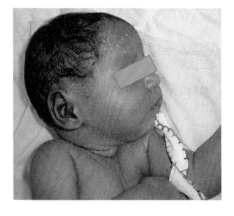

FIGURE 4.7A A newborn baby had this tiny vesicular rash all over the body that was more prominent on the forehead, neck, upper chest, and flexures. The child was afebrile and clinically well.

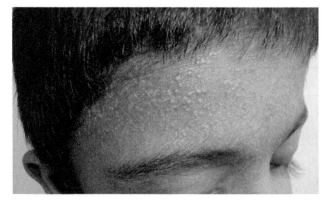

FIGURE 4.7B A 9-year-old boy with miliaria crystallina.

Based on the case description and Figure 4.7a, what are your differential diagnoses?

1. Miliaria crystallina
2. Viral exanthem

MILIARIA

Diagnosis

Miliaria crystallina

Discussion

This is a common acute or subacute skin condition that arises due to the occlusion or disruption of eccrine sweat ducts in hot humid conditions, resulting in a leakage of sweat. There are three forms of miliaria due to the different levels at which occlusion occurs: in miliaria crystallina, the obstruction is very superficial, within the stratum corneum; in miliaria rubra (prickly heat), the changes include keratinization of the intraepidermal part of the sweat duct; and in miliaria profunda, there is rupture of the duct at the level of or below the dermal–epidermal junction. So the leakage of sweat occurs into the epidermis (miliaria crystallina and miliaria rubra) or dermis (miliaria profunda).

Clinical features of the three types of miliaria differ (Coulson & Wilson, 2016).

- *Miliaria crystallina:* Clear, thin-walled vesicles, 1–2 mm in diameter without an inflammatory areola, are usually symptomless and develop in crops, mainly on the trunk. The vesicles soon rupture, and are followed by superficial, branny desquamation.
- *Miliaria rubra (prickly heat):* This is the commonest form in hot humid climates. These lesions commonly appear on the occluded skin of the neck, groins, and axillae, but also occur elsewhere. The lesions are uniformly minute erythematous papules that produce intense discomfort in the form of an unbearable pricking sensation.
- *Miliaria profunda:* This nearly always follows repeated attacks of miliaria rubra, and is uncommon even in the tropics. The affected skin is covered with pale, firm papules 1–3 mm across, especially on the body, but sometimes also on the limbs. There is no itching or discomfort from the lesions; therefore they are easily missed.

The most important complications of miliaria are secondary infection and disturbance of heat regulation. Infection may present as impetigo. In most cases of miliaria rubra the changes are reversible if further sweating is avoided, but permanent damage to the sweat duct may occur, especially after miliaria profunda.

Investigations

This is a clinical diagnosis.

Management

- The only really effective prevention or treatment for miliaria is avoidance of further sweating. Avoidance of excessive clothing, friction from clothing, excessive use of soap, and contact of the skin with irritants will reduce recurrences. (Palaniappan et al., 2023)
- Controlling local environment (removing excess bedding, using fans, air conditioning) and cooling the skin (damp compresses, cool showers) are important.
- Calamine lotion is effective for the relief of discomfort.
- Topical antibiotics may be used if there is secondary infection and mild topical steroids if extensive and/or itchy.

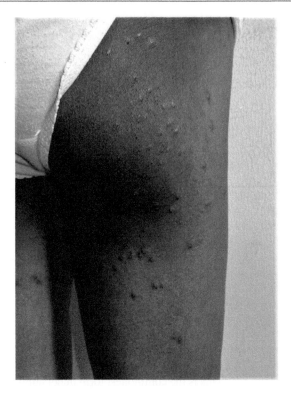

FIGURE 4.8 Itchy hyperpigmented papules on exposed parts of the body in a 7-year-old girl. In tropical climate young children wear minimal clothes during the hot humid daytime.

Based on the case description and Figure 4.8, what are your differential diagnoses?

1. Papular urticaria
2. Scabies

PAPULAR URTICARIA

Diagnosis

Papular urticaria

Discussion

Papular urticaria arises as a result of a hypersensitivity reaction to insect bites, mostly mosquitoes, ants, and ticks in the tropics. It usually appears as itchy papules and papulovesicles, most frequently on exposed areas of the extremities. In the tropics, children usually stay bare-trunked due to the hot humid climate, and papules may extend to buttocks and trunk as in this case. Secondary bacterial infection is common. Reactivation of old lesions by new insect bites causes diagnostic confusion because most parents do not accept multiple insect bites. This is thought to arise from circulating insect antigen-stimulating cutaneous T cells in previously sensitized sites (Higgins & Glover, 2016).

Investigations

This is a clinical diagnosis.

Management

The treatment of papular urticaria includes topical steroids and systemic antihistamines, but response is usually limited, and the condition will only be controlled if insect bites can be avoided (Kamath, 2020). Wearing full-coverage clothes from 4:00 pm onwards, and use of mosquito repellents during that time, are important to avoid mosquito bites which is the commonest cause in tropical climate.

Children eventually outgrow this disease at 10–12 years of age, probably through desensitization after multiple arthropod exposures. However, rarely this may extend to adulthood, and then it may persist long term.

Refractory cases may benefit from subcutaneous specific immunotherapy (Collado Chagoya et al., 2022).

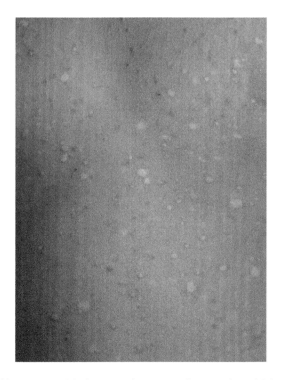

FIGURE 4.9 A 6-year-old boy came with these erythematous tiny papules which spontaneously heal leaving post-inflammatory hypopigmentation for more than 5 months. These lesions were asymptomatic and the child was clinically well.

Based on the case description and Figure 4.9, what are your differential diagnoses?

1. Pityriasis lichenoides chronica
2. Guttate psoriasis

PITYRIASIS LICHENOIDES CHRONICA (PLC)

Diagnosis

Pityriasis lichenoides chronica (PLC)

Discussion

The cause of pityriasis lichenoides is unknown. It occurs most frequently in children and young adults.

Clinically, pityriasis lichenoides is divided into two main conditions: pityriasis lichenoides chronica (PLC) and pityriasis lichenoides et varioliformis acuta (PLEVA). The distinction between PLC and PLEVA is based on clinical morphology and histology rather than disease course. Both PLEVA and PLC last on average 18 months with an episodic course.

The characteristic lesion in PLC is a small, firm, reddish brown papule 3–10 mm in diameter. An adherent "mica-like" scale can be detached by gentle scraping to reveal a shining brown surface—a distinctive diagnostic feature. Over 3 or 4 weeks, the papule flattens and the scale separates spontaneously to leave a pigmented macule, which gradually fades leaving post-inflammatory hypopigmentation (Elbendary et al., 2022). Eruption is generalized but an isolated acral form and segmental forms have been reported. Constitutional symptoms such as fever, headache, malaise, and arthralgia are absent in PLC, features that differentiate from PLEVA (Lane & Parker, 2010).

In PLEVA constitutional symptoms such as fever, headache, malaise, and arthralgia may precede or accompany the onset of lesions. The initial lesion is an oedematous pink papule that undergoes central vesiculation and haemorrhagic necrosis. The vesicles may be small or so large that they may appear bullous. New lesions are often asymptomatic. These heal with scarring.

Secondary syphilis needs to be excluded, especially if the palms and soles are involved or if there are mucosal lesions.

Investigations

Skin biopsy for histopathology

Management

Management of both PLC and PLEVA is similar. Management is almost same in both children and adults. Topical corticosteroids may improve symptoms and healing of lesions but do not alter the course of the disease (Child & Whittaker, 2016).

Management of PLC in Children

- *First line:* Topical steroids/topical tacrolimus ointment
- *Second line:* Antibiotics (erythromycin) (in adults phototherapy is used: broad-/narrow-band UVB, PUVA)
- *Third line:* Methotrexate, ciclosporin, dapsone (in adults acitretin [acitretin plus PUVA] or UVA-1 can be used)

Management of PLEVA in Children

- *First line:* Oral antibiotics (erythromycin)
- *Second line:* Phototherapy (broad-/narrow-band UVB) (in adults acitretin plus PUVA is used)
- *Third line:* Systemic corticosteroids, methotrexate, ciclosporin, dapsone (in adults UVA-1 is used)

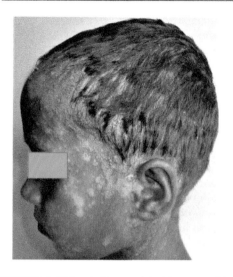

FIGURE 4.10A A 6-year-old girl came with generalized non-itchy scaly rash for 4 months. Scales were marked on the scalp. She did not have a history of similar rash before.

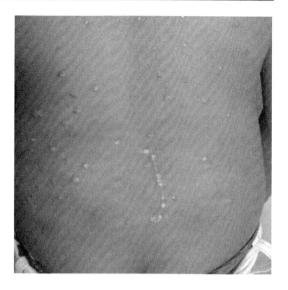

FIGURE 4.10B Guttate psoriasis and Koebner phenomenon (the lesions occurring in sites of cutaneous trauma and old scars).

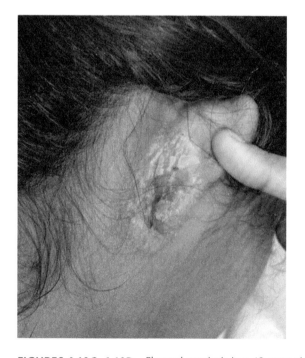

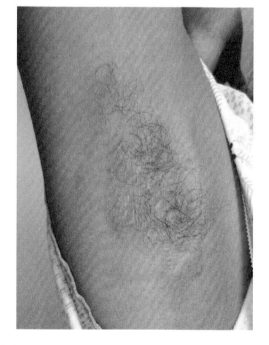

FIGURES 4.10C, 4.10D Flexural psoriasis in a 12-year-old girl. Note the minimal scaling in flexures.

Based on the case description and Figure 4.10a, what are your differential diagnoses?

1. Seborrhoeic dermatitis
2. Psoriasis

PSORIASIS

Diagnosis

Psoriasis

Discussion

Psoriasis is common in children. In infancy, napkin psoriasis with or without disseminated lesions is the most frequent form, presenting with well-defined erythema devoid of scales. At this site, psoriasis must be differentiated from irritant contact dermatitis or nappy rash, and infantile seborrhoeic dermatitis. The napkin area is frequently the first site affected under the age of 2 years. Guttate psoriasis (Figure 4.10b) is more frequent in children than adults, particularly under the age of 12 years.

In older children, plaque psoriasis is the most frequent presentation (Burden & Kirby, 2016). The most characteristic lesions in plaque psoriasis consist of silvery scaly, indurated plaques which are remarkably well demarcated from unaffected skin. Erythema or redness is minimal or absent in darker-skinned individuals (Mallawaarachchi, 2021). When severity of plaque psoriasis is assessed using PASI (Psoriasis Area Severity Index), since the erythema is 0 or 1 in darker skin, PASI score gives false security in equally affected darker-skinned persons than in white-skinned patients.

Although it is stated that psoriasis appears to be more common in countries that are further from the equator and in white people, it is very common in Sri Lanka (a tropical country with brown-skinned people), too. There are two peak ages of incidence, the first occurring between 16 and 22 years and the second between 57 and 62 years of age. Plaque psoriasis is the most common type of psoriasis, accounting for about 80–90% of all cases. Psoriasis commonly presents over the extensor surfaces and scalp. The amount of scaling may be minimal in partially treated disease, and in the flexures (Figure 4.10c, d).

Investigations

This is a clinical diagnosis.

Management

Management of psoriasis should be assessed individually. Treatment depends upon many variables including age, gender, occupation, personality, general health, intelligence, and resources, as well as the type, extent, site, duration, and natural history of the disease.

The children are best managed with less cumbersome, less toxic therapies: emollients, diluted topical corticosteroids, topical vitamin D analogues. Systemic methotrexate or acitretin may be tried in extensive plaque psoriasis in older children that do not respond to topical therapies or in pustular psoriasis.

"Proactive therapy" is a recent approach in childhood-onset psoriasis that would help to prevent the severity of flare-ups, thus improving the quality of life and avoiding poor performances in school (Dhar & Srinivas, 2022; Lavaud & Mahé, 2020)

Proactive Topical Therapy

It is useful in mild types of psoriasis in which plaques recur at the same sites.

- Gradual withdrawal over several months to prevent frequent relapses (topical corticosteroids)
- Weekend therapy (topical corticosteroids and calcipotriol)
- On-demand therapy—early treatment of first symptom of flare effectively prevents further episodes (topical corticosteroids and calcipotriol)

Proactive Systemic Therapy

- *Maintenance of remission with minimum effective dose:* After initial phase of active treatment, systemic drug is either tapered to lowest maintenance dose (nonbiologics) or interval of intake is spaced (biologics).
- *Weekend therapy:* The minimal effective dose is given on weekends (ciclosporine).
- *Intermittent therapy:* It is the reintroduction of drug during initial stages of relapse (ciclosporine/etanercept).

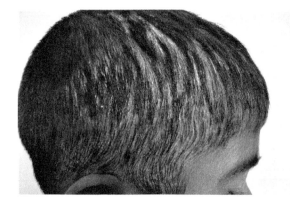

FIGURE 4.11   A 10-year-old boy complained of his scaly scalp that does not respond to anti-dandruff therapies prescribed by his family physician. On examination, thick scales adherent to the scalp and hair were noted.

Based on the case description and Figure 4.11, what are your differential diagnoses?

1. Tinea amiantacea
2. Scalp psoriasis
3. Dandruff

TINEA AMIANTACEA

Diagnosis

Pityriasis amiantacea/Tinea amiantacea

Discussion

Pityriasis amiantacea refers to a scaling pattern on the scalp in which the scales overlap like tiles on a roof. The matted scale is attached to the underlying hair shafts. Some consider pityriasis amiantacea to be a form of severe psoriasis whilst others consider this a pattern that can be attributable to a range of causes such as seborrhoeic dermatitis, eczema, lichen simplex, and psoriasis. Pityriasis amiantacea can be localized or may involve the whole scalp. It is most common in children and young adults (Amorim & Fernandes, 2016).

Investigations

This is a clinical diagnosis.

Managements

Manage as scalp psoriasis: apply topical coal tar (4–6%) and salicylic (4%) ointment nocte to the scalp, and wash it the next morning using an antifungal shampoo; this should be done daily until complete clearance, then continue the same once or twice a week as maintenance therapy.

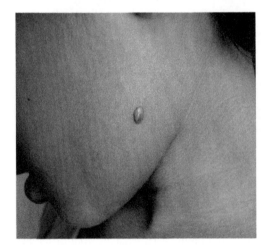

FIGURE 4.12   A 6-year-old girl presented with an asymptomatic lump for more than 6 months.

Based on the case description and Figure 4.12, what are your differential diagnoses?

1. Juvenile xanthogranuloma
2. Basal cell carcinoma (not seen in darker-skinned children)
3. Cystic lump

XANTHOGRANULOMA

Diagnosis

Juvenile xanthogranuloma

Discussion

This is a benign proliferative disorder of histiocytes occurring in early infancy and childhood that regresses spontaneously within 1–5 years. Single lesions are the most common, but multiple lesions, ranging from a few to hundreds, may occur. Giant JXG is defined as a lesion greater than 2 cm in diameter. Most systemic lesions undergo spontaneous resolution in 1–5 years; however, ocular and CNS involvement may lead to significant complications. In ocular involvement, acute hyphaema, glaucoma, and blindness may occur while seizures, ataxia, increased intracranial pressure, subdural effusions, developmental delay, diabetes insipidus, and other neurological deficits are complications of CNS lesions (Tran et al., 2016).

Management

- Since juvenile xanthogranuloma resolve spontaneously, they do not require treatment.
- Reassure the parents, and parents need to be warned that occasionally resolution may result in a scar.
- In single and accessible lesions, surgical excision is curative.

REFERENCES

Amorim GM, Fernandes NC (2016). Pityriasis amiantacea: A study of seven cases. *Anais Brasileiros de Dermatologia*;91(5):694–6. doi: 10.1590/abd1806-4841.20164951.

Aróstegui Aguilar J, Loidi L, Hiltun I, et al. (2022). Pediatric genital lichen sclerosus: A case series of 11 girls. *Anales del Sistema Sanitario de Navarra* 18;45(3):e1014 (Spanish). doi: 10.23938/ASSN.1014.

Bunker CB, Porter WM (2016). Dermatoses of the male genitalia. In Christopher G, Jonathan B, Tanya B, Robert C, Daniel C, eds. *Rook's Textbook of Dermatology*, 9th edn. Hoboken: Wiley-Blackwell, 111.13p.

Burden AD, Kirby B (2016). Psoriasis and related disorders. In Christopher G, Jonathan B, Tanya B, Robert C, Daniel C, eds. *Rook's Textbook of Dermatology*, 9th edn. Hoboken: Wiley-Blackwell, 35.1p.

Child LF, Whittaker SJ (2016). Lymphocytic infiltrates. In Christopher G, Jonathan B, Tanya B, Robert C, Daniel C, eds. *Rook's Textbook of Dermatology*, 9th edn. Hoboken: Wiley-Blackwell, 135.3p.

Collado Chagoya R, Hernández-Romero J, Velasco-Medina AA, Velázquez-Sámano G (2022). Pilot study: Specific immunotherapy in patients with papular urticaria by Cimex lectularius. *European Annals of Allergy and Clinical Immunology*;54(6):258–64. doi: 10.23822/EurAnnACI.1764-1489.215.

Corazza M, Schettini N, Zedde P, Borghi A (2021). Vulvar lichen sclerosus from pathophysiology to therapeutic approaches: Evidence and prospects. *Biomedicines* 3;9(8):950. doi: 10.3390/biomedicines9080950.

Coulson IH, Wilson NJE (2016). Disorders of the sweat glands. In Christopher G, Jonathan B, Tanya B, Robert C, Daniel C, eds. *Rook's Textbook of Dermatology*, 9th edn. Hoboken: Wiley-Blackwell, 94.12p.

Dennin MH, Stein SL, Rosenblatt AE (2018) Vitiligoid variant of lichen sclerosus in young girls with darker skin types. *Pediatric Dermatology*;35(2):198–201. doi: 10.1111/pde.13399.

Dhar S, Srinivas SM (2022). Psoriasis in pediatric age group. *The Indian Journal of Dermatology*;67(4):374–80. doi: 10.4103/ijd.ijd_570_22.

Elbendary A, Abdel-Halim MRE, Youssef R, et al. (2022). Hypopigmented lesions in pityriasis lichenoides chronica patients: Are they only post-inflammatory hypopigmentation? *Australasian Journal of Dermatology* 2022;63(1):68–73. doi: 10.1111/ajd.13746.

Grattan CEH, Radia DH (2016). Mastocytosis. In Christopher G, Jonathan B, Tanya B, Robert C, Daniel C, eds. *Rook's Textbook of Dermatology*, 9th edn. Hoboken: Wiley-Blackwell, 46.1p.

Higgins EM, Glover MT. (2016) Dermatoses and haemangiomas of infancy. In Christopher G, Jonathan B, Tanya B, Robert C, Daniel C, eds. *Rook's Textbook of Dermatology*, 9th edn. Hoboken: Wiley-Blackwell, 117.3p.

Joshi TP, Duvic M (2022). Granuloma annulare: An updated review of epidemiology, pathogenesis, and treatment options. *The American Journal of Clinical Dermatology*;23(1):37–50. doi: 10.1007/s40257-021-00636-1.

Kamath S, Kenner-Bell B (2020). Infestations, bites, and insect repellents. *Pediatric Annals* 1;49(3):e124–31. doi: 10.3928/19382359-20200214-01. PMID: 32155278.

Kannangara AP (2021). Lichen planus and lichenoid dermatoses. In Ranawaka RR, Kannangara AP, Karawita A, eds. *Atlas of Dermatoses in Pigmented Skin*. Singapore: Springer, pp. 497–502. doi: 10.1007/978-981-15-5483-4_25.

Lane TN, Parker SS (2010). Pityriasis lichenoides chronica in black patients. *Cutis*;85(3):125–9.

Lavaud J, Mahé E (2020). Proactive treatment in childhood psoriasis. *Annales de Dermatologie et de Vénéréologie*;147(1):29–35. doi: 10.1016/j.annder.2019.07.005.

Lewis F (2016). Dermatoses of the female genitalia. In Christopher G, Jonathan B, Tanya B, Robert C, Daniel C, eds. *Rook's Textbook of Dermatology*, 9th edn. Hoboken: Wiley-Blackwell, 112.6p.

Mallawaarachchi K (2021). Psoriasis. In Ranawaka RR, Kannangara AP, Karawita A, eds. *Atlas of Dermatoses in Pigmented Skin*. Singapore: Springer, pp. 91–106. doi: 10.1007/978-981-15-5483-4_5.

Melin A, Bouchereau S, Guelimi R, et al. (2022). Safety and efficacy of high-dose clobetasol propionate 0.05% in cutaneous lichen planus. *The Journal of Dermatology* 28. doi: 10.1111/1346-8138.16689.

Oyama N, Hasegawa M (2022). Lichen sclerosus: A current landscape of autoimmune and genetic interplay. *Diagnostics* (Basel) 6;12(12):3070. doi: 10.3390/diagnostics12123070.

Özkur E, Aksu EK, Gürel MS, Savaş S (2019). Comparison of topical clobetasol propionate 0.05% and topical tacrolimus 0.1% in the treatment of cutaneous lichen planus. *Postepy Dermatology and Allergology*;36(6):722–6. doi: 10.5114/ada.2019.91423.

Palaniappan V, Sadhasivamohan A, Sankarapandian J, Karthikeyan K (2023). Miliaria crystallina. *Clinical and Experimental Dermatology* 24:llad032. doi: 10.1093/ced/llad032.

Piguet V, Breathnach SM, Le Cleach L (2016) Lichen planus and lichenoid disorders. In Christopher G, Jonathan B, Tanya B, Robert C, Daniel C, eds. *Rook's Textbook of Dermatology*, 9th edn. Hoboken: Wiley-Blackwell, 37.1p.

Ranawaka RR (2021a). Hypopigmented mycosis fungoides. In Ranawaka RR, Kannangara AP, Karawita A, eds. *Atlas of Dermatoses in Pigmented Skin*. Singapore: Springer, pp. 921–37. doi: 10.1007/978-981-15-5483-4_49.

Ranawaka RR (2021b). Precursors of skin carcinoma. In Ranawaka RR, Kannangara AP, Karawita A, eds. *Atlas of Dermatoses in Pigmented Skin*. Singapore: Springer, pp. 971–88. doi: 10.1007/978-981-15-5483-4_49.

Ranawaka RR, Abeygunasekara PH, De Silva MVC (2011). Hypopigmented mycosis fungoides in type V skin: A report of 5 cases. *Case Reports in Dermatological Medicine*, Article ID 190572, doi:10.1155/2011/190572 PMID: 23198169

Sandru F, Petca RC, Costescu M, et al. (2021) Cutaneous mastocytosis in childhood-update from the literature. *Journal of Clinical Medicine* 2;10(7):1474. doi: 10.3390/jcm10071474.

Tiano R, Krase IZ, Sacco K (2022). Updates in diagnosis and management of paediatric mastocytosis. *Current Opinion in Allergy and Clinical Immunology* 3. doi: 10.1097/ACI.0000000000000869.

Tran TH, Pope E, Weitzman S (2016). Cutaneous histiocytoses. In Christopher G, Jonathan B, Tanya B, Robert C, Daniel C, eds. *Rook's Textbook of Dermatology*, 9th edn. Hoboken: Wiley-Blackwell, 136.12p.

van Geel N, Speeckaert R (2016). Acquired pigmentary disorders. In Christopher G, Jonathan B, Tanya B, Robert C, Daniel C, eds. *Rook's Textbook of Dermatology*, 9th edn. Hoboken: Wiley-Blackwell, 88.32p.

Veronesi G, Virdi A, Leuzzi M, et al. (2021) Vulvar vitiligo and lichen sclerosus in children: A clinical challenge. *Pediatric Dermatology*;38(5):1012–9. doi: 10.1111/pde.14771.

Wain EM, Orchard GE, Whittaker SJ, et al. (2003). Outcome in 34 patients with juvenile-onset mycosis fungoides: A clinical, immunophenotypic, and molecular study. *Cancer* 15;98(10):2282–90.

Wang J, Khachemoune A (2018). Granuloma annulare: A focused review of therapeutic options. *The American Journal of Clinical Dermatology*;19(3):333–44. doi: 10.1007/s40257-017-0334-5.

Hypo- and Hyperpigmentary Disorders in Children with FST 5

5

Ajith P. Kannangara

INTRODUCTION

This chapter discusses 7 common hypo- and hyperpigmentary dermatoses we encounter in children with brown skin (Fitzpatrick skin type V/FST 5) using clinical photographs. These are discussed based on clinical photographs and easy-to-read question-and-answer format. They are ashy dermatosis, fixed drug eruption, morphoea, pityriasis alba, post-inflammatory hypopigmentation, progressive macular hypomelanosis, and vitiligo.

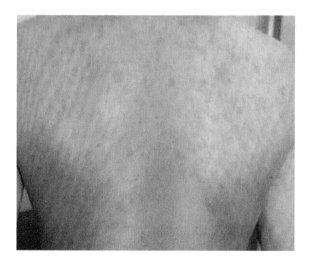

FIGURE 5.1 A 17-year-school boy came with 9 months' history of gradually increasing multiple macular blackish pigmentations of his body involving chest, back of the chest, arms, neck, and face, which poorly responded to "whitening creams" which he had been using for 7–8 weeks.

DOI: 10.1201/9781003321507-5

Based on the clinical history and Figure 5.1, what is your differential diagnosis?

1. Ashy dermatosis
2. Lichen planus pigmentosus
3. Occupational dermatosis with hyperpigmentation
4. Drug-related dermatoses
5. Universal acquired melanosis

ASHY DERMATOSIS

Diagnosis

Ashy dermatosis

Discussion

Ashy dermatosis and erythema dyschromicum perstans are two distinct entities in terms of the extent of the inflammation, albeit on the same spectrum of pigment disorders. Ashy dermatosis is an idiopathic hypermelanotic disorder characterized by bluish grey macules, mostly symmetrical, usually affecting the face, arms, neck, and trunk in healthy individuals. Dark-coloured individuals are most affected in their second decade of life. Mucosa is rarely involved (Chakrabarti & Chattopadhyay, 2012).

Erythema dyschromicum perstans is characterized by erythema occurring on the border of the pigmented macules. The authors have never seen an inflammatory phase with erythema in darker-skinned patients. Therefore, ashy dermatosis is a more appropriate term in our brown-skinned patients.

Investigations

Skin biopsy and histopathology; the active border in erythema dyschromicum perstans lesions shows vacuolar degeneration of the basal cells. In both erythema dyschromicum perstans and ashy dermatosis, the epidermis contains much pigment, and there is pigmentary incontinence. The dermal vessels are sleeved with an infiltrate of lymphocytes and histiocytes, and there are pigment incontinence and many melanophages in the deep dermis (Numata et al., 2015).

Management

There is no consistently effective treatment. The initial erythematous phase tends to settle after several months. The pigmentation is persistent with a tendency to extend gradually over years. The drug of choice is clofazimine (van Geel & Speeckaert, 2016).

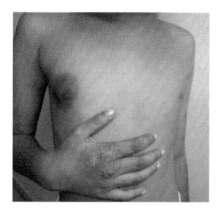

FIGURE 5.2A A 9-year-old girl came with an itchy scaly lesion on the right hand for 6-month duration. The mother had noticed that this had been enlarging over the period, and on and off becomes itchy and scaly. She also complained of a hyperpigmented patch on the right breast which is enlarging progressively, too. (Photographed by Dr. Ranthilaka R. Gammanpila.)

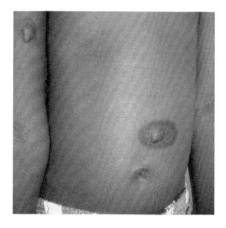

FIGURE 5.2B Fixed drug eruption in acute stage. Acute blisters appear on top of previous hyperpigmented patches whenever exposed to the same allergen; the existing lesion progressively enlarges and new blisters appear on fresh sites. (Photographed by Dr. Ranthilaka R. Gammanpila.)

Based on the case description and Figure 5.2a, what are your differential diagnoses?

1. Fixed drug eruption
2. Bullous lichen planus
3. Drug-induced pemphigus
4. Lichenoid drug eruption
5. Discoid eczema

FIXED DRUG ERUPTION

Diagnosis

Fixed drug eruption

Discussion

Fixed drug eruption is an adverse reaction of exposure to drugs such as sulfonamides, barbiturates, carbamazepine, or tetracycline. Lesions appear on the skin/mucosa, with predilection for lips, palms, soles, or genitalia, 1–8 h post exposure. There is a tendency of recurrence in the same area or involving several sites, in case of re-exposure of the offending drug. It is characterized by solitary or multiple lesions, oedematous, red-dusky, round to oval, well circumscribed, with a diameter of 1–5 cm and occasional central blistering. Lesions may show mild pruritus. Oral lesions may present different morphologies including bullous, erosive, or aphthous, and affect mainly the hard palate or dorsum of the tongue. Perianal and genital areas may be affected. Lesions heal with residual hyperpigmentation (Özkaya, 2013; Shiohara, 2009).

Investigations

This is a clinical diagnosis.

Management

It has a good prognosis; after drug discontinuation lesions resolve spontaneously. Treatment options include antihistamines and topical or systemic corticosteroids.

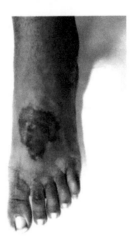

FIGURE 5.3A A 14-year-old boy presented with 2 months' history of asymptomatic slow-growing atrophic plaque on his left foot.

Based on the clinical history and Figure 5.3a, what is your differential diagnosis?

1. Morphoea
2. Extragenital lichen sclerosus
3. Morpheaform basal cell carcinoma
4. Post-inflammatory hyperpigmentation

MORPHOEA

Diagnosis

Morphoea

Discussion

Plaque-type morphoea is the most frequent type of morphoea and lesions appear as well-circumscribed indurated plaques with pigmentary changes, typically confined to the epidermis and dermis. Clinical features include round- or oval-shaped areas of hard and shiny skin, most frequently appearing on the trunk and proximal extremities. The morphology of the lesions is dependent on the disease duration. In the initial stage, the lesions usually appear erythematous. A characteristic violaceous halo can be seen around the plaque, which corresponds to the inflammatory phase of morphoea. When the disease progresses, indurated hairless plaques develop at the centre of these lesions. This leads to the appearance of a yellow-white or ivory-coloured sclerotic plaque with an erythematous or violaceous border called "lilac ring". In some cases, sclerosis may be limited or even absent, with dyspigmentation or atrophy being the predominant feature (Fett et al., 2011).

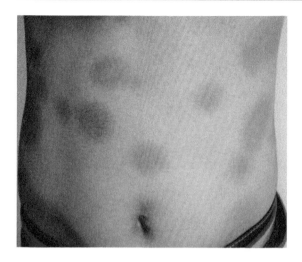

FIGURE 5.3B Disseminated plaque morphoea in a 13-year-old girl. (Photographed by Dr. Ranthilaka R. Gammanpila.)

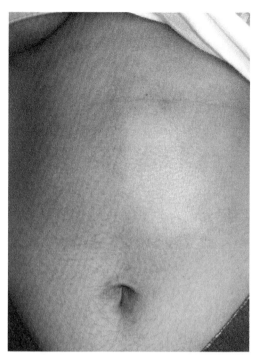

FIGURE 5.3C An 11-year-old girl presented with this solitary skin change which had appeared over a month. Skin biopsy confirmed morphoea. Note the erythematous ring surrounding the yellowish white central sclerotic area (sclerotic phase in morphoea). This phase is rarely observed in darker skin.

Commonly, patients present to us with well-demarcated hyperpigmented macules (Figure 5.3b), which if untreated become bound-down, hyperpigmented, thickened, shiny, waxy macules. There may be loss of hair and absent sweating. Erythematous, oedematous, inflammatory phase, or yellowish white sclerotic phase described in white skin is rarely observed in brown skinned patients (Figure 5.3c). Central sclerotic area surrounded by an erythematous to violaceous so-called "lilac ring" (sclerotic phase) has rarely observed in brown-skinned patients. This could be due to the darker skin that obscure erythema or violaceous colour.

Cases of lichen sclerosus occurring in conjunction with morphoea are now well documented (Figure 5.3d).

Investigations

This is a clinical diagnosis but histopathology is performed for confirmation. In the early active inflammatory phase, newer lesions demonstrate a lymphocytic infiltrate, with a variable number of plasma cells and eosinophils. As lesions evolve, the numbers of inflammatory cells are reduced as collagen bundles thicken and skin sclerosis increases in the later fibrotic phase. The depth of involvement differs in different clinical types; in plaque morphoea they may be limited to the dermis, whereas in linear and deep types they may extend beyond the skin and into the underlying fascia, muscle, and bone.

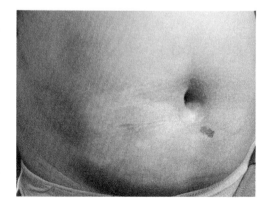

FIGURE 5.3D Co-existing of morphoea (dark brown colour) and lichen sclerosus (whitish colour) in a 9-year-old boy. He had multiple morphoea lesions but only one LS lesion. Skin biopsy was performed from both lesions for confirmation. (Photographed by Dr. Ranthilaka R. Gammanpila.)

Management

Treatment is best utilized in the initial stage of morphea to reduce inflammation and prevent progression of the disease. Moderate- to high-potency topical corticosteroids, tacrolimus, calcipotriol, and phototherapy (UVA-1) are used for the treatment (Fett, 2012). While the course of the disease and treatment response is difficult to predict, in most patients the lesions will spontaneously involute after 3–5 years.

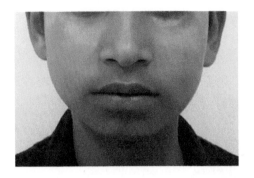

FIGURE 5.4   This schoolboy came with a history of asymptomatic hypopigmented macular areas on his face for few weeks.

Based on the clinical history and Figure 5.4, what is your differential diagnosis?

1. Pityriasis alba
2. Tinea versicolor
3. Photodermatitis
4. Vitiligo
5. Post-inflammatory hypopigmentation

PITYRIASIS ALBA

Diagnosis

Pityriasis alba

Discussion

Pityriasis alba is a common form of mild eczematous childhood dermatitis seen in atopic individuals. This term is derived from its fine scaly appearance (pityriasis) in conjunction with the pallor of the affected patches of skin (alba). Pityriasis alba is characterized by ill-defined, dry patches with hypopigmentation and fine scale. Patches usually range from 0.5 to 2 cm in diameter but may be as large as 4 cm or even more. There is a typical distribution in exposed areas such as the cheeks, shoulders, or upper trunk. Affected areas may appear more conspicuous during warmer weather seasons due to sun exposure of juxtaposed normal skin. Dry scaling may be exaggerated during the winter months.

Investigations

This is mainly a clinical diagnosis. Skin scraping for fungal study, Wood's lamp examination, and dermatoscopy may be helpful to exclude differential diagnoses.

Management

Pityriasis alba is usually a self-limiting condition and lesions often improve with emollients or mild topical corticosteroids.

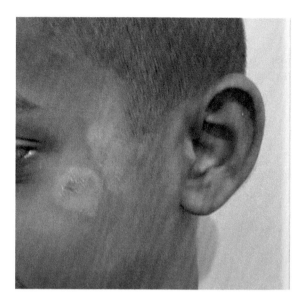

FIGURE 5.5   This schoolboy presented with a mildly itchy scaly hypopigmented macular area on his face for few weeks.

Based on the clinical history and Figure 5.5, what is your differential diagnosis?

1. Post-inflammatory hypopigmentation (following polymorphic light eruption)
2. Pityriasis alba
3. Tinea versicolor
4. Vitiligo

POST-INFLAMMATORY HYPOPIGMENTATION

Diagnosis

Post-inflammatory hypopigmentation

Discussion

Post-inflammatory hypopigmentation is a common, acquired dermatologic entity that denotes decreased or absent skin pigmentation following a wide variety of cutaneous inflammatory or infectious insults. It is thought that inflammation results in altered melanogenesis and transfer of melanosomes from melanocytes to keratinocytes, leading to hypomelanosis. Clinical features are more obvious in tanned or darkly pigmented individuals but does occur in all races. The hypopigmentation typically presents as macules or patches that are confined to areas of previous photodamage insult (Vachiramon, 2011).

Investigations

This is a clinical diagnosis. Examination under Wood's light can help accentuate lesions, but this is clearly apparent in darker skin and Wood's light examination is unnecessary.

Management

When the underlying disorder is treated, post-inflammatory hypopigmentation will gradually resolve over weeks to months. Complete re-pigmentation of the affected tissues is observed unless there had been loss of functional melanocytes.

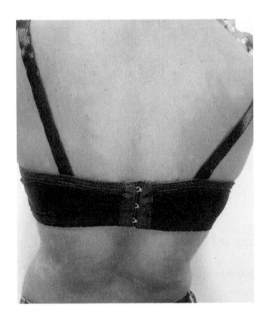

FIGURE 5.6 A 17-year-old girl came with a history of gradually progressing asymptomatic hypopigmented macula area involving the trunk for 3 years.

Based on the clinical history and Figure 5.6, what is your differential diagnosis?

1. Progressive macular hypomelanosis (PMH)
2. Tinea versicolor
3. Post-inflammatory hypopigmentation
4. Hypopigmented mycosis fungoides

PROGRESSIVE MACULAR HYPOMELANOSIS

Diagnosis

Progressive macular hypomelanosis

Discussion

Progressive macular hypomelanosis is an acquired disorder of hypopigmentation most frequently seen in young, dark-skinned individuals either living in or originally from tropical climates. There is a female predominance. It presents with ill-defined, hypopigmented macules primarily affecting the back of the trunk, chest, and abdomen. The macules may coalesce along the midline to form large hypopigmented patches. There are no overlying scales and lesions are usually asymptomatic (Relyveld et al., 2007).

Investigations

This is a clinical diagnosis.

Wood's lamp examination of affected areas shows coral red follicular fluorescence. Porphyrin production by *Propionibacterium* species has been described and it would be the most probable reason for this. Skin biopsy and histopathological examination are performed in difficult cases to differentiate it from hypopigmented mycosis fungoides.

Management

This condition generally resolves spontaneously after several years. Treatment with topical clindamycin, benzoyl peroxide, and phototherapy (both UVA and narrow-band UVB) has been shown to be effective (Duarte et al., 2010).

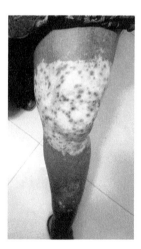

FIGURE 5.7A A 17-year-old obese type 1 diabetic patient came with 11 months' history of asymptomatic rapidly growing hypopigmented area on her left leg.

Based on the clinical history and Figure 5.7a, what is your differential diagnosis?

1. Vitiligo
2. Post-inflammatory hypomelanosis
3. Extragenital lichen scleroses et atrophicus

VITILIGO

Diagnosis

Vitiligo

Discussion

Vitiligo is caused by an absence of functional melanocytes secondary to melanocytic destruction. The latest accepted leading theory hypothesizes that there is an autoimmune process with alterations in cellular and humoral immunity. Other etiologic theories include inherent melanocyte alterations, cytotoxic mechanisms by local metabolites, and oxidative stress-induced destruction. Vitiligo is characterized by well-circumscribed areas of depigmented macules and patches. Most predilection sites are the fingers, wrists, axillae, groin, genitalia, and periocular and perioral areas. All areas of the body may be involved, and the development of new lesions on traumatized skin or following trauma may occur (Koebner phenomenon). It is mainly classified into segmental and non-segmental patterns of distribution. The segmental form is defined by one or more macules or patches involving a unilateral segment of the body. Non-segmental is defined by involvement of more than one segment or diffuse involvement of the body. Extensive involvement which involves 80–90% of the body surface and is usually preceded by the generalized form which has gradually evolved is defined as vitiligo universalis (Ezzedine et al., 2012, 2015).

Investigations

This is a clinical diagnosis.

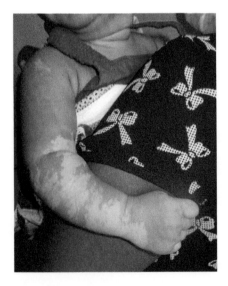

FIGURE 5.7B Dermatomal vitiligo since birth in a 7-month-old baby girl. (Photographed by Dr. Ranthilaka R. Gammanpila.)

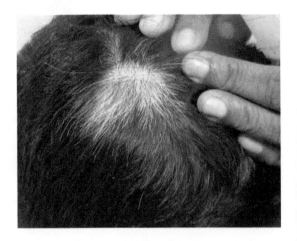

FIGURE 5.7C A 6-year-old boy presented with premature grey hair which was progressing. Examination revealed a localized area of white hair where underlying scalp skin was depigmented. This is vitiligo on the scalp and associated poliosis or leukotrichia. (Photographed by Dr. Ranthilaka R. Gammanpila.)

Pathological examination reveals decreased or absent melanocytes and/or melanin in the stratum basalis upon routine haematoxylin and eosin staining. Immunohistochemical staining with Melan-A and HMB-45 may aid in the evaluation of epidermal melanocytes. A Fontana–Masson melanin stain may also be utilized. A perivascular lymphocytic infiltrate has been described in early lesions.

Management

There are a few good prognostic indicators including new onset of disease, young age, and central location of lesions such as face, neck, and trunk. Poor prognostic indicators include family history, Koebner phenomenon, acral distribution, and segmental disease (Gawkrodger et al., 2008)

No definitive cure is currently available. Topical steroids, calcineurin inhibiters, and Janus kinase inhibiters are used in mild to moderate cases. Oral steroids are indicated to hold or suppress the rapidly spreading vitiligo. Phototherapy including PUVA (Psoralens and UVA), UVB, and Excimer laser are other forms of treatment with variable success. Immunosuppressive therapy and photodynamic therapy may also be utilized. For extensive disease, depigmentation therapy with monobenzone, 4-(Benzyloxy)phenol, or hydroquinone cream may be attempted on their remaining pigmented skin (Dillon et al., 2017).

REFERENCES

Chakrabarti N, Chattopadhyay C (2012). Ashy dermatosis: A controversial entity. *The Indian Journal of Dermatology*;57(1):61–2.

Dillon AB, Sideris A, Hadi A, Elbuluk N (2017). Advances in vitiligo: An update on medical and surgical treatments. *The Journal of Clinical and Aesthetic Dermatology*;10(1):15–28.

Duarte I, Della Nina B, Gordiano M, et al. (2010). Progressive macular hypomelanosis: An epidemiological study and therapeutic response to phototherapy (treatment). *Anais Brasileiros de Dermatologia*;85(5):621–4.

Ezzedine K, Eleftheriadou V, Whitton M, Van Geel N (2015). Vitiligo. *Lancet*;386(9988):74–84.

Ezzedine K, Lim HW, Suzuki T, et al. (2012). Revised classification/nomenclature of vitiligo and related issues: The vitiligo global issues consensus conference. *Pigment Cell & Melanoma Research*;25(3):E1–3.

Fett N, Werth VP (2011). Update on morphea: Part I. Epidemiology, clinical presentation, and pathogenesis. *The Journal of the American Academy of Dermatology*;64(2):217–28.

Fett NM (2012). Morphea: Evidence-based recommendations for treatment. *The Indian Journal of Dermatology, Venereology and Leprology*;78(2):135–41.

Gawkrodger DJ, Ormerod AD, Shaw L, et al (2008) Guideline for the diagnosis and management of vitiligo. *The British Journal of Dermatology*;159(5):1051–76.

Numata T, HaRada K, Tsuboi R, Mitsuhashi Y (2015). Erythema dyschromicum perstans: Identical to ashy dermatosis or not? *Case Reports in Dermatology*;7(2):46–50.

Özkaya E (2013). Oral mucosal fixed drug eruption: Characteristics and differential diagnosis. *The Journal of the American Academy of Dermatology*;69(2):e51–8.

Relyveld GN, Menke HE, Westerhof W (2007). Progressive macular hypomelanosis: An overview. *The American Journal of Clinical Dermatology*;8(1):13–9.

Shiohara T (2009). Fixed drug eruption: Pathogenesis and diagnostic tests. *Current Opinion in Allergy and Clinical Immunology*;9(4):316–21.

Vachiramon V, Thadanipon K (2011). Postinflammatory hypopigmentation. *The Journal of Clinical & Experimental Dermatology*;36(7):708–14.

van Geel N, Speeckaert R (2016). Acquired pigmentary disorders. In Griffiths C, Barker J, Bleiker T, Chalmers R, Creamer D, eds. *Rook's Textbook of Dermatology*, vol. 88, 9th edn. Oxford: Wiley-Blackwell, pp. 13–33.

Hair and Nail Disorders in Children with FST 5

6

Ajith P. Kannangara

INTRODUCTION

This chapter discusses 11 common hair and nail dermatoses we encounter in children with brown skin (Fitzpatrick skin type V/FST 5) using clinical photographs. These are discussed based on clinical photographs and easy-to-read question-and-answer format. They are acute paronychia, alopecia areata, anagen effluvium, Beau's line, frictional alopecia, onychomadesis, longitudinal melanonychia, nail lichen planus, pincer nail (trumpet nail), telogen effluvium, and trichotillosis (hair pulling disorder).

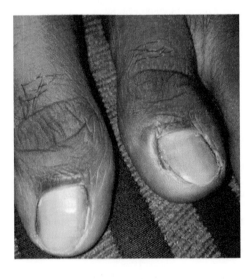

FIGURE 6.1 A 16-year-old boy presented with a 6-week history of discolouration of lateral nail plate with on and off painful swelling of nail folds. He had a habit of frequent washing of his legs from the garden tap while playing in the garden.

Based on the clinical history and Figure 6.1, what is your differential diagnosis?

1. Acute bacterial paronychia
2. Chronic paronychia
3. Onychocryptosis

DOI: 10.1201/9781003321507-6

ACUTE BACTERIAL PARONYCHIA

Diagnosis

Acute bacterial paronychia

Discussion

Acute bacterial paronychia may occur secondary to trauma, offending shoe gear, faulty biomechanics, and toenail anatomy. The most common infective agent is *Staphylococcus aureus*, but *Streptococcus*, *Pseudomonas*, and some Gram-negative bacteria have also been cultured. The presence of anaerobic bacteria is seen in the presence of oral inoculation. Purulence can tract underneath the nail and cause elevation of the nail from the nail plate. Clinical features of true acute bacterial paronychia may or may not be in the presence of an ingrowing toenail. If an ingrowing nail is present, the nail acts as a foreign body and is therefore a nidus for infection. However, bacterial colonization without nail incurvation is common. Regardless of causes, patients present with discomfort and clinical signs of localized infection.

Investigations

This is a clinical diagnosis.

Management

Treatment is based on the aetiology of the acute paronychia and includes conservative treatments with soaking, trimming back the offending nail border, nail bracing, taping, change of shoe gear, removal of the offending nail border in cases of ingrowing nail, resection of small wedge in acute cases, partial or complete nail avulsion with chemical matrixectomy for chronic and refractory cases, and broad-spectrum antibiotics.

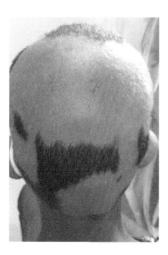

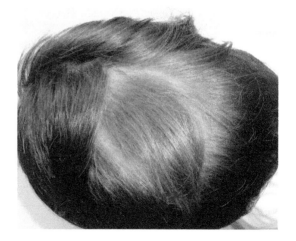

FIGURE 6.2A   A 17-year-old girl presented with an 8-month history of gradually losing her hair on multiple sites without responding to home remedies and native treatments.

FIGURE 6.2B   Alopecia areata: during the regrowth phase, hair may be de-pigmented, but hair pigmentation recovers completely within months. (Photographed by Dr. Ranthilaka R. Gammanpila.)

Based on the clinical history and Figure 6.2a, what is your differential diagnosis?

1. Alopecia areata (early alopecia totalis)
2. Trichotillomania
3. Traction alopecia

ALOPECIA AREATA

Diagnosis

Alopecia areata

Discussion

Alopecia areata is an autoimmune process that develops specifically against hair follicles (Petukhova et al., 2010). It is one of the most common reasons for non-scarring hair loss and one of the most prevalent autoimmune disorders. This condition is characterized by a disfiguring inflammatory condition perturbing hair follicles and nail structure. It mostly appears insidiously with patches of hair loss which may increase in size, coalesce, and progress to affect whole scalp or body. "Exclamation point hairs" (a type of dystrophic hair in the periphery of the lesion) are pathognomonic for the diagnosis of alopecia areata. Atopic dermatitis, allergic rhinitis, asthma, thyroid disease, vitiligo, diabetes mellitus, Down syndrome, collagen vascular diseases, and nail changes have been reported in association with this disease (Goh et al., 2006; Sharma et al., 1996).

Investigations

Diagnosis is usually clinical.

In pathological study, peribulbar inflammation is frequently seen adjacent to lesions around hair follicles in anagen phase. The involved follicles re-enter anagen. In early stages, reduction in the size of hair follicles below the level of sebaceous gland is seen along with preservation of the part above the sebaceous gland. The sebaceous glands are also preserved. The smaller hair follicles in the anagen phase are mitotically active and can produce a normal inner root sheath. The cortex of hair shafts is incompletely keratinized.

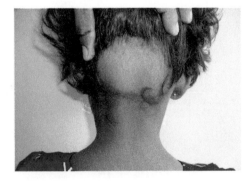

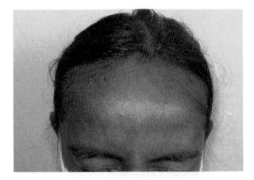

FIGURE 6.2C Alopecia areata: ophiasis pattern in a 9-year-old girl. The prognosis is less favourable in childhood onset and in ophiasis pattern. (Photographed by Dr. Ranthilaka R. Gammanpila.)

FIGURE 6.2D Reverse ophiasis pattern of alopecia areata in a 10-year-old girl. (Photographed by Dr. Ranthilaka R. Gammanpila.)

Management

The severity of alopecia areata can be predicted by the age of onset; childhood onset disorder has a poor prognosis, particularly in men.

Intralesional, topical, or systemic corticosteroids, anthralin, methotrexate, azathioprine, ciclosporin, sulfasalazine, minoxidil, adalimumab, tofacitinib, and ruxolitinib are used for its treatment.

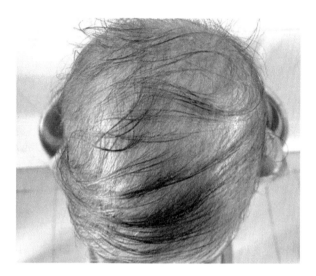

FIGURE 6.3 A 12-year-old girl who was recently diagnosed to have acute leukaemia came with sudden severe loss of hair for two-week duration.

Based on the case description and Figure 6.3, what is your differential diagnosis?

1. Anagen effluvium
2. Telogen effluvium
3. Androgenetic alopecia
4. Alopecia areata (diffuse)

ANAGEN EFFLUVIUM

Diagnosis

Anagen effluvium

Discussion

Anagen effluvium is the abrupt hair loss involving the anagen phase hairs. It is caused by impairment of the mitotic or metabolic activity of hair follicles. Radiotherapy and chemotherapy with agents such as alkylating agents, antimetabolites, and mitotic inhibitors are its common etiologic factors. Because 75–80% of scalp hairs are in the anagen phase, an extensive portion of the scalp is affected in this condition. It is classified as a non-scarring alopecia with intact follicular ostia and no evidence of erythema, scaling, and pigmentation. It begins within days to 2–3 weeks after the offending insult like chemotherapy that results in near-complete hair loss by 2–3 months. The severity of hair loss varies from person to person and is dependent on factors like the kind of chemotherapeutic agent, its dose, duration of the treatment, and its administration route. Affected patients have 10–20% of their hair remaining after the culprit insult (Kanwar & Narang, 2013).

Investigations

Diagnosis is mainly clinical.

Management

This condition is usually reversible, hence wearing a wig until full hair regrowth is the best coping strategy for affected persons.

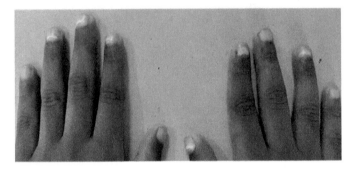

FIGURE 6.4A A 7-year-old girl presented with 2-week history of destruction and shedding of her nails. She had a history of hand foot and mouth disease 7 weeks ago.

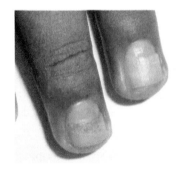

FIGURE 6.4B Onychomadesis (closer view) in an infant following hand foot and mouth disease.

Based on the clinical history and Figure 6.4a, what is your differential diagnosis?

1. Beau's line and onychomadesis
2. Onychomycosis
3. Onychodystrophy
4. Habit-tic deformity

BEAU'S LINE

Diagnosis

Beau's line and onychomadesis

Discussion

Beau's lines are transverse depressions in the nail plate which originate within the matrix and progress distally as the nail grows. They occur following a stressful event that temporarily interrupts nail growth. Beau's lines are described as the most common and least specific nail change in systemic diseases. The margin is parallel to the lunula when the cause is internal, and it is more apparent on thumb and great toe-nails. If there is complete inhibition of nail growth for around 2 weeks, Beau's line will reach maximum depth resulting in onychomadesis (Braswell et al., 2015).

Onychomadesis results from complete toxicity of the matrix and can present with shedding of the nail or a proximal sulcus that splits the nail plate into two parts. This condition is an extreme expression of Beau's lines, and the causes are the same (Damevska et al., 2015).

Investigation

Pathological study is not applicable, and diagnosis is mainly history and clinical appearance.

Management

Depending on the cause, its management includes treatment of the underlying cause or waiting for the nail to grow gradually.

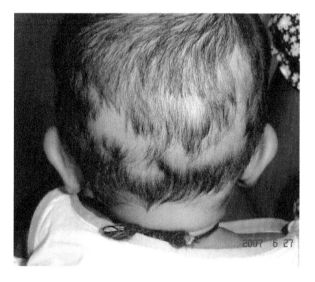

FIGURE 6.5   A 4-month-old baby was brought with patchy hair loss on the back of the scalp. (Photographed by Dr. Ranthilaka R. Ranawaka.)

Based on the clinical history and Figure 6.5, what is your differential diagnosis?

1. Frictional alopecia
2. Diffuse alopecia areata
3. Alopecia induced by nutritional deficit

FRICTIONAL ALOPECIA

Diagnosis

Frictional alopecia

Discussion

Transient neonatal hair loss encompasses the very common phenomenon of neonatal occipital alopecia and development of bald patches in other locations. Healthy babies have been observed to develop alopecic oval patches, most notably in the occiput, during the first 2 months of life. Friction was the presumed cause of transient neonatal hair loss, with the occiput particularly affected due to supine sleeping positions creating friction between the back of their head and the surface they're blissfully snoozing away on. This causes their delicate hair to tangle and break and is known as pressure or friction alopecia.

Management

Friction alopecia or pressure alopecia has a benign course with no accompanying symptoms, and the hair spontaneously regrows.

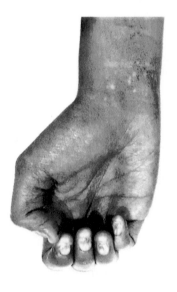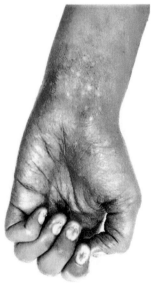

FIGURE 6.6 A 17-year-old girl presented with a 4-month history of destruction and thinning of her nails. She had a history of pigmented ulcerated buccal mucosa 6 to 7 months ago.

Based on the clinical history and Figure 6.6, what is your differential diagnosis?

1. Nail lichen planus
2. Nail psoriasis
3. Darier disease-related nail change
4. Onychomycosis

NAIL LICHEN PLANUS

Diagnosis

Nail lichen planus

Discussion

Nail changes are seen in 10% of patients with disseminated lichen planus (Wagner et al., 2013). Fingernails are more affected. Although aetiology of the disease is unclear, an autoimmune reaction in which CD8+ T lymphocytes attack basal keratinocytes leading to cell death has been suggested. Factors such as viral or bacterial antigens, drugs, and physical causes can trigger the autoimmune attack. Clinically, thinning of the nail plate and longitudinal ridging are the first hints of an isolated involvement of the nails. Characteristic nail changes include dorsal pterygium unguis. The trachyonychia is evident by roughness of the nail plate, a grey discolouration of the nail, and loss of transparency of the nail. The disease can develop on several nails simultaneously (Tosti et al., 1993; Nakamura et al., 2013).

Investigation

Diagnosis is mainly clinical.

Management

Nail lichen planus may present with variable progression depending on the timing of the diagnosis. Treatments include topical and systemic corticosteroids; other topical agents including tacrolimus, pimecrolimus, ciclosporine, and retinoids; and systemic agents such as biologic agents, metronidazole, and thalidomide.

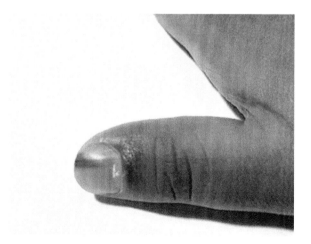

FIGURE 6.7 An 18-month-old boy presented with a 6-week history of longitudinal dark discolouration of right thumb nail, and his parents were worried about this pigmentary change.

Based on the clinical history and Figure 6.7, what is your differential diagnosis?

1. Longitudinal melanonychia
2. Exogenous substances (dirt, tar)
3. Subungual hematoma
4. Subungual melanoma

LONGITUDINAL MELANONYCHIA

Diagnosis

Longitudinal melanonychia

Discussion

Longitudinal melanonychia, also known as melanonychia striata, is a pigmented band in the nail plate which results from deposition of melanin via nail matrix melanocytes. It is usually common in darkly pigmented individuals. Its aetiology includes racial melanonychia, pregnancy, trauma, inflammatory states (lichen planus and psoriasis), iatrogenic (medication) and systemic diseases (Addison's disease), and syndrome-associated melanonychia (e.g., Laugier–Hunziker, Peutz–Jeghers, and Touraine syndromes). It is characterized by brown or black longitudinal bands of hyperpigmentation within the nail plate and originates in the nail matrix and extends to the distal edge of the nail plate. It can involve single or multiple nails depending on the etiology. Extension of pigment into periungual area is referred to as Hutchinson's sign and may also be an important clinical indicator of malignancy (Jefferson & Rich, 2012; Metzner et al., 2015).

Management

The majority of melanonychia has a benign cause and does not warrant treatment. Management of underlying systemic disease or discontinuation of the offending substance may be enough to decrease nail hyperpigmentation.

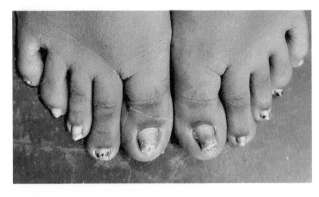

FIGURE 6.8 A 14-year-old girl presented with a one-year history of discolouration and thickening of several of her toenails which she was unable to trim as she wanted.

Based on the clinical history and Figure 6.8, what is your differential diagnosis?

1. Pincer nail (trumpet nail)
2. Ingrown toenail
3. Psoriasis
4. Onychomycosis

PINCER NAIL (TRUMPET NAIL)

Diagnosis

Pincer nail (trumpet nail)

Discussion

Pincer nail, also known as the trumpet nail, is a severely curved nail that progresses distally and is not the same as an ingrown nail. It can be hereditary or acquired. It may be painful. It is hypothesized that pincer nails may either be caused by the lack of ground reaction force on the digit or by an increase in the automatic curvature force. A pincer nail is a result of transverse over-curvature of the nail plate that increases distally along the longitudinal axis. It often affects the great toenail but can affect any nail. It may appear because of nail psoriasis, underlying tumour, ill-fitting shoes, and other biomechanical issues of the foot (Baran et al., 2001).

Management

Recurrence is high with conservative therapies (trimming, debridement, bracing) if the underlying disorder is not addressed. To target the underlying disorder, a surgical procedure such as the inverted T addresses the boney osteophyte and flattens out the nail bed.

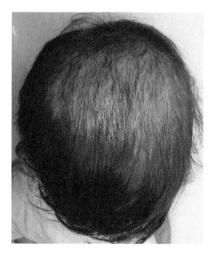

FIGURE 6.9 A 7-year-old girl presented with recent-onset excessive hair loss on the vertex. Detailed direct inquiry revealed that she had dengue fever 3 months ago, and was hospitalized for a week. She was otherwise a healthy child. (Photographed by Dr. Ranthilaka R. Gammanpila.)

Based on the clinical history and Figure 6.9, what is your differential diagnosis?

1. Acute telogen effluvium
2. Anagen effluvium (excluded from the medical history)
3. Trichotillosis (excluded from the history, and vertex is not an easily accessible area)
4. Androgenic alopecia
5. Diffuse alopecia areata

TELOGEN EFFLUVIUM

Diagnosis

Telogen effluvium

Discussion

Telogen effluvium is an increase in the shedding of telogen club hairs due to premature termination of the anagen phase of the hair cycle. There are two types: acute and chronic, depending on the time of onset (Malkud, 2015).

Acute telogen effluvium is an acute-onset scalp hair loss that occurs 2–3 months after a triggering event such as a high fever, surgical trauma, sudden starvation, or haemorrhage. However, in two thirds of cases, triggering factors are not identified. This does not produce total baldness. If the trigger is not repeated, spontaneous complete regrowth occurs within 3–6 months.

If the insult is prolonged or repeated, shedding can continue. Chronic diffuse telogen hair loss refers to telogen hair shedding persisting for longer than 6 months. Identified causes for chronic telogen effluvium are thyroid disorders (both hyper- and hypothyroidism), profound iron deficiency anaemia, acrodermatitis enteropathica, acquired zinc deficiency, and malnutrition.

Investigations

Trichoscopy in experienced hands may help to differentiate from other mimics.

Management

Acute telogen effluvium is self-limited. In chronic cases, underlying factors should be identified and dealt with.

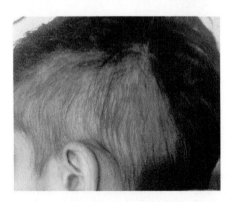

FIGURE 6.10 A 7-year-old boy who was recently admitted to primary school was brought by the parents with unilateral sudden severe loss of hair for a 3-week duration.

Based on the case description and Figure 6.10, what is your differential diagnosis?

1. Trichotillosis
2. Alopecia areata
3. Lupus erythematous
4. Fungal infection

TRICHOTILLOSIS (HAIR PULLING DISORDER)

Diagnosis

Trichotillosis

Discussion

Trichotillosis or hair pulling disorder is an impulse control disorder with repetitive pulling of hair causing a non-scarring alopecia with hairs in different lengths. The scalp, eyelashes, and eyebrows are the most commonly affected areas and typically, the hairs are short, irregular, broken, and distorted. The diagnosis is mainly established on clinical grounds with very specific trichoscopy signs such as V sign, flame hairs, tulip hair, hook hairs, hair powder, and follicular micro-haemorrhages. More frequent but less specific signs include decreased capillary density, broken hairs, black spots, trichoptilosis, short vellus, yellow spots, and exclamation mark hairs (Ankad et al., 2014; Barroso et al., 2017).

This may associate with trichorhizophagia (hair root alone is eaten) or trichophagia (the whole hair is eaten) (Sandoz et al., 2008).

Management

Psychotherapy and selective serotonin reuptake inhibitors are also helpful. The prognosis is better when the disorder is diagnosed early, and treatment begins early.

REFERENCES

Ankad BS, Naidu MV, Beergouder SL, Sujana L (2014). Trichoscopy in trichotillomania: A useful diagnostic tool. *International Journal of Trichology*;6(4):160–3.
Baran R, Haneke E, Richert B (2001). Pincer nails: Definition and surgical treatment. *Dermatologic Surgery*;27(3):261–6.
Barroso Lal, Sternberg F, Souza Mnife, Nunes GJB (2017). Trichotillomania: A good response to treatment with N-acetylcysteine. *Anais Brasileiros de Dermatologia*;92(4):537–9.
Braswell MA, Daniel CR 3rd, Brodell RT (2015). Beau lines, onychomadesis, and retronychia: A unifying hypothesis. *Journal of the American Academy of Dermatology*;73(5):849–55
Damevska K, Gocev G, Pollozahani N, et al (2015). Onychomadesis following cutaneous vasculitis. *Acta Dermatovenerologica Croatica*;25(1):77–9.
Goh C, Finkel M, Christos PJ, Sinha AA (2006). Profile of 513 patients with alopecia areata: Associations of disease subtypes with atopy, autoimmune disease, and positive family history. *Journal of the European Academy of Dermatology and Venereology*;20(9):1055–60.

Jefferson J, Rich P (2012). Melanonychia. *Dermatology Research and Practice* 2012: 952186

Kanwar AJ, Narang T (2013). Anagen effluvium. *The Indian Journal of Dermatology, Venereology and Leprology*;79(5):604–12.

Malkud S (2015). Telogen effluvium: A review. *Journal of Clinical and Diagnostic Research*;9(9): WE01–3.

Metzner MJ, Billington AR, Payne WG (2015). Melanonychia. *Eplasty*;15:ic48 (eCollection 2015).

Nakamura R, Broce AA, Palencia DP, et al (2013). Dermatoscopy of nail lichen planus. *The International Journal of Dermatology*;52(6):684–7.

Petukhova L, Duvic M, Hordinsky M et al. (2010). Genome-wide association study in alopecia areata implicates both innate and adaptive immunity. *Nature*;466(7302):113–7.

Sandoz A, Koenig T, Kusnir D, Tausk F (2008). Psychocutaneous diseases. In Wolff K, Goldsmith L, Katz S, Gilchrest B, Paller AS, Leffell D, eds. *Fitzpatrick's Dermatology in General Medicine*, 7th edn. New York: McGraw-Hill Companies.

Sharma VK, Dawn G, Kumar B (1996). Profile of alopecia areata in northern India. *The International Journal of Dermatology*;35:22–7.

Tosti A, Peluso AM, Fanti PA, Piraccini BM (1993). Nail lichen planus: Clinical and pathologic study of twenty-four patients. *The Journal of the American Academy of Dermatology*;28(5 Pt 1):724–30.

Wagner G, Rose C, Sachse MM (2013). Clinical variants of lichen planus. *Journal Der Deutschen Dermatologischen Gesellschaft*;11(4):309–19.

Genetic Dermatoses in Children with FST 5

7

Ranthilaka R. Gammanpila

INTRODUCTION

This chapter discusses 9 common genetic dermatoses we encounter in children with brown skin (Fitzpatrick skin type V/FST 5) using 13 clinical photographs. These are discussed based on clinical photographs and easy-to-read question-and-answer format. They are acrodermatitis enteropathica (zinc deficiency), anetoderma, cutis laxa, ectodermal dysplasia, epidermolysis bullosa, lipoid proteinases, Marfan syndrome, neurofibromatosis, and tuberous sclerosis.

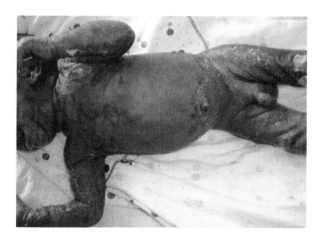

FIGURE 7.1 A newborn pre-term baby in a premature baby unit was referred with the pictured skin rash. The child was irritable and had low birth weight. The baby had been treated with intravenous antibiotics without improvement.

Based on the case description and Figure 7.1, what are your differential diagnoses?

1. Zinc deficiency syndrome (acrodermatitis enteropathica)
2. Epidermolysis bullosa
3. Toxic shock syndrome
4. Staphylococcal scalded skin syndrome (SSSS)

DOI: 10.1201/9781003321507-7

ACRODERMATITIS ENTEROPATHICA OR ZINC DEFICIENCY

Diagnosis

Zinc deficiency syndrome

Discussion

Premature infants are at high risk for developing zinc deficiency. Not only do premature infants have higher metabolic demands, they also have inadequate stores since maternal transfer of zinc typically occurs during the last 10 weeks of gestation.

Acrodermatitis enteropathica is an inherited disorder (autosomal recessive) affecting the intestinal absorption of zinc. Zinc is a co-factor for over 200 enzymes. The skin, intestine, and immune system are most severely affected because of their rapid cell turnover. The classic triad of zinc deficiency is diarrhoea, alopecia, and a periorificial and acral skin eruption (Searle et al., 2022).

In full-term breastfeeding babies the symptoms start after weaning from the breast, and at 4–10 weeks of age in formula-fed babies. Patients present with apathy or irritability and a rash around the mouth and anus and on the hands and feet. Erythema progresses to vesicles, bullae, pustules, desquamation, and crusting. There is alopecia and frequently blepharitis, conjunctivitis, and photophobia. Infections are common. Wound healing is poor and many patients have diarrhoea and growth faltering. Other cutaneous findings include angular cheilitis, paronychia, delayed wound healing, and vitiligo-like hypopigmentation (Chu et al., 2016; Zou et al., 2023).

Investigations

This is a clinical diagnosis. The serum zinc concentration is usually low but can be normal (<70 µg/L fasting). It is easier to undertake a trial of zinc therapy: patients respond within 24–48 hours.

Management

Patients respond to oral zinc sulfate within a few days. The normal dose is 2–3 mg/day in childhood up to 3 years of age; 5 mg/day for children 4–8 years of age; and 8 mg/day for children 9–14 years of age. Adolescents and adults require 8–13 mg/day. Patients with acrodermatitis enteropathica require lifelong supplementation with 3 mg/kg/day of elemental zinc (50 mg elemental zinc per 220 mg zinc sulfate) (Glutsch et al., 2019).

Monitoring for copper deficiency should be undertaken.

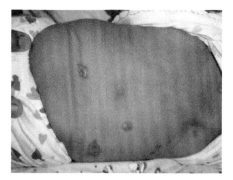

FIGURE 7.2 A newborn baby had these skin patches on the trunk since birth. These were asymptomatic circumscribed areas of slack skin.

Based on the case description and Figure 7.2, what are your differential diagnoses?

1. Anetoderma (macular atrophy)
2. Congenital syphilis and scarring
3. Birth injuries and scarring

ANETODERMA

Diagnosis

Anetoderma

Discussion

The term anetoderma (*anetos*: slack) refers to a circumscribed area of slack skin associated with a loss of dermal substance on palpation and a loss of elastic tissue on histological examination. Primary anetoderma is strongly associated with antiphospholipid syndrome with or without features of systemic lupus. Secondary anetoderma has been reported in association with many inflammatory skin conditions such as urticaria, Stevens–Johnson syndrome, B- and T-cell lymphoma, tuberculosis and leprosy, urticaria pigmentosa, pityriasis versicolor, and granuloma annulare. Anetoderma is common among 20–40-year-old adults, and uncommon in infancy (Lovell, 2016; Cook & Puckett, 2022).

In this child, the mother had chickenpox during the pregnancy and intrauterine chickenpox causing these multiple atrophic scars was the only identifiable cause.

Investigations

Histopathology confirms the clinical diagnosis. The fragmentation and disappearance of elastic tissue is the essential change, beginning superficially in the subpapillary zone and extending downwards.

Management

No specific treatment exists. In the case of secondary anetoderma, treatment should be directed against underlying disease or infections.

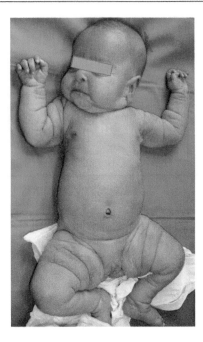

FIGURE 7.3 This 7-month-old baby was brought with recurrent chest infections. She died a few months later due to respiratory complications.

Based on the case description and Figure 7.3, what are your differential diagnoses?

1. Inherited cutis laxa
2. Wrinkly skin syndrome: skin changes are limited mainly to the abdomen, hands, and feet
3. Acquired cutis laxa: this may rarely develop at any age but often follows an inflammatory process or an associated disorder such as antiphospholipid syndrome or SLE
4. Ehlers–Danlos syndrome (EDS): the skin is hyperextensible but not lax, and it recoils quickly
5. Pseudo xanthoma elasticum (PXE): the skin may be lax, but it is yellowish and the face is usually spared. It is distinguished histologically by the presence of calcification.

CUTIS LAXA

Diagnosis

Inherited cutis laxa

Discussion

Cutis laxa is a group of conditions in which the skin lacks elasticity leading to a loose, wrinkly, and prematurely aged appearance. It is variably associated with connective tissue problems as a result of loss, disorganization, or fragmentation of elastic tissues in other organs, notably the lungs, cardiovascular system, joints, and gastrointestinal and genito-urinary systems. Cutis laxa is very rare, with an estimated incidence of one in 4 million.

A number of different genes and chromosome abnormalities have been identified as causing different phenotypes. Patients with autosomal dominant cutis laxa have lax skin and a prematurely aged appearance with onset between childhood and early adulthood, as well as gastrointestinal diverticula, inguinal hernias, emphysema, aortic aneurysm, and aortic or mitral valve prolapse. Autosomal recessive cutis laxa comprises severe forms with life-threatening complications and death occurring between infancy and young adulthood usually from cardiorespiratory compromise. X-linked cutis laxa affects males only (Mohamed et al., 2014; Burrows, 2016).

Investigations

This is a clinical diagnosis. Histologically, there is loss and fragmentation of elastic tissue in the dermis.

Management

Routine management is indicated for complications such as refractive errors, emphysema, hip dislocation, inguinal hernias, and seizures.

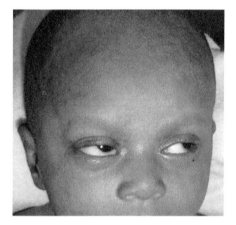

FIGURE 7.4   This 5-month-old baby boy was brought due to sparse hair on the scalp and the eyebrow. Note hypotrichosis, reduced eyebrows and eyelashes in this child. The mother had also noted the lack of sweating in the child making him uncomfortable and irritable in the hot humid climate.

Based on the case description and Figure 7.4, what are your differential diagnoses?

1. Hypohidrotic or anhidrotic ectodermal dysplasia
2. Sjogren syndrome with symptomatic sicca syndrome
3. Other forms of ectodermal dysplasia with immunodeficiency or deafness

ECTODERMAL DYSPLASIA

Diagnosis

Hypohidrotic or anhidrotic ectodermal dysplasia

Discussion

Ectodermal dysplasias, a large group of heterogeneous inheritable conditions, are characterized by congenital defects in two or more ectodermal structures: hair (trichodysplasia), teeth (dental defects), nails (onychodysplasia), or sweat glands (dyshidrosis).

X-linked hypohidrotic or anhidrotic ectodermal dysplasia is the most common of the ectodermal dysplasias. The disorder is characterized by hypotrichosis with fine, slow-growing scalp and body hair, sparse eyebrows, hypohidrosis, nail anomalies, and hypodontia. Peg-shaped primary and secondary teeth are typical. Decreased sweating leads to heat intolerance and enhances dryness of the skin with episodes of hyperpyrexia, which may result in seizures and neurological damage. Due to a lower body surface area ratio, thermoregulation is most problematic in infants and young children who may experience recurrent bouts of fever as high as 42°C. Heatstroke is the most common cause of death in patients with anhidrotic ectodermal dysplasia within the first years of life. Anhidrotic ectodermal dysplasia is associated with mortality rates as high as 21% (Itin, 2016; Wright et al., 2022).

Investigations

This is a clinical diagnosis. Radiographs of the jaws may reveal dental hypoplasia or aplasia. Histology shows missing or reduced sweat glands and also reduced sebaceous glands. The epidermis is thin with flattening of the rete ridges. About 80% of obligate female carriers of X-linked HED have distinct dental abnormalities including absent permanent teeth and small or peg-shaped teeth. 7.5.4 Management

Early diagnosis is vital to avoid life-threatening complications induced by hyperthermia and infections.

Patients should avoid hot places and extensive physical activity without cooling devices and special clothes. Patients should drink cool liquids in warm environments. Cooling the body with wet clothing and cool drinks is the only efficient way of treating hyperthermia.

Orthodontic intervention is necessary, particularly for language development.

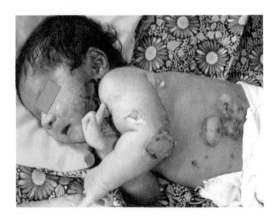

FIGURE 7.5 This newborn baby developed blisters and ulcers on frictional sites a few hours after birth. This is the third child of these parents whose elder two children had had similar skin manifestations and had died within a few months.

Based on the case description and Figure 7.5, what are your differential diagnoses?

1. Epidermolysis bullosa (junctional EB type)
2. Staph impetigo
3. Toxic epidermal necrolysis (TEN)

EPIDERMOLYSIS BULLOSA

Diagnosis

Epidermolysis bullosa

Discussion

Epidermolysis bullosa comprises a group of genetically determined skin fragility disorders characterized by blistering of the skin and mucosae following mild mechanical trauma (*mechanobullous diseases*). They are classified into many clinical subtypes depending on the clinical manifestations and histological level of skin involvement (basal, suprabasal, junctional). Clinical manifestations depend on the severity of skin involvement: mild localized frictional blisters (EB simplex) to extensive lesions with mucosal involvement (junctional EB and dystrophic EB).

Clinically, the mildest form is **EB simplex** which is again subdivided into basal and suprabasal variants, that manifest as more than 12 distinct clinical disorders. **Localized EB simplex** is the most common type of EB; inheritance is autosomal dominant in which frictional blisters appear on the soles and palms.

Almost all clinical variants of **junctional EB** are characterized by autosomal recessive inheritance and by blister formation at the level of the lamina lucida. Conventionally, junctional EB is divided into two main categories: generalized and localized, each of which has a number of subtypes.

Dystrophic EB is characterized by skin fragility, blistering, scarring, nail dystrophy, and milia formation. Mucosal involvement is common, and erosions and scarring can affect the mouth, oesophagus, genitalia, and anus. There are several subtypes depending on the genetic inheritance (autosomal dominant or recessive) and other organ involvement (McGrath, 2016).

Differential diagnosis

Differentiating EB from non-EB, or one form of EB from another, can be very difficult, especially in the neonatal period. Other causes of blistering diseases should be considered: infective (staphylococcal scalded skin syndrome, bullous impetigo, neonatal herpes infection); inflammatory (erythema toxicum neonatorum, urticaria pigmentosa); autoimmune (pemphigus or pemphigoid gestationis), and metabolic (acrodermatitis enteropathica, aminoaciduria).

Investigations

Skin biopsy for histopathology and immunofluorescence: less than 12 h old, a sample of non-blistered skin that has been gently rubbed to produce a mild erythema is preferable, because this will usually contain a cleavage plane. The main objective of skin biopsy is to establish the level of blistering or tissue separation. Because the diagnostic signs are mostly seen in and around the dermal–epidermal junction, shave biopsy samples are preferable to thicker specimens. The samples should be immediately immersed in suitable fixative for electron microscopy or in Michel's transport medium for immunofluorescence.

Management

At present there is no curative treatment for any form of EB, and the mainstay of clinical management is based on protection and avoidance of provoking factors, and symptomatic management. Topical gene therapy and topical calcipotriol ointment have been studied on wound healing (Gurevich et al., 2022; Bolton, 2022).

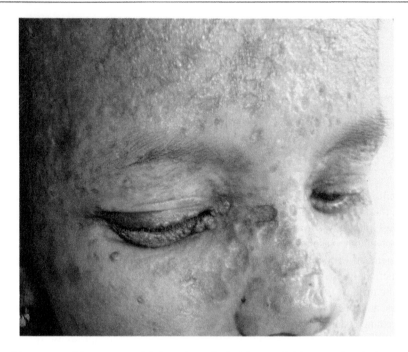

FIGURE 7.6   This 12-year-old came complaining of patchy hair loss and thinning of scalp hair. Note acneiform, pock-like scars on the face, characteristic "beaded" papules along the margins of the eyelids, and diminished eyelashes.

Based on the case description and Figure 7.6, what are your differential diagnoses?

1. Lipoid proteinosis
2. Erythropoietic protoporphyria (this causes waxy papules and depressed scars but the scars are confined to sun-exposed skin)
3. Xanthomatosis
4. Amyloidosis
5. Lichen myxoedematosus
6. Myxoedema with hoarseness (in early infancy)

LIPOID PROTEINOSIS

Diagnosis

Lipoid proteinosis

Discussion

Lipoid proteinosis is a rare autosomal recessive disorder, characterized by infiltration of hyaline material into the skin, oral cavity, larynx, and internal organs (Morris, 2016). This presents in early infancy with hoarseness. The vocal cords are thickened, with nodules here and on the epiglottis. The lips, pharynx, soft palate, uvula, and tonsils develop yellow-white submucous infiltrates. The tongue is enlarged and firm with infiltrates on its undersurface. The first skin lesions are often blisters in early childhood. Acneiform, pock-like scars appear on the face. Characteristic "beaded" papules are present along the margins of the eyelids. There may be loss of eyelashes or patchy alopecia due to scalp involvement. Infiltration of the skin can cause waxy papules, hyperkeratosis, or warty plaques, which may become darker with time. These lesions may affect the palms or backs of the hands, forehead, or elbows. Epilepsy and psychiatric problems occur in a number of patients and may be associated with intracranial calcification (Burrows, 2016; Hamada, 2002).

Investigations

The dermis is thickened and the upper dermis contains large deposits of extracellular hyaline material that stains strongly with periodic acid–Schiff (PAS).

Management

Symptomatic management only. Microlaryngoscopy and dissection of the vocal cords can be successful.
   Dermabrasion, chemical skin peeling, blepharoplasty, and carbon dioxide laser therapy may be helpful.

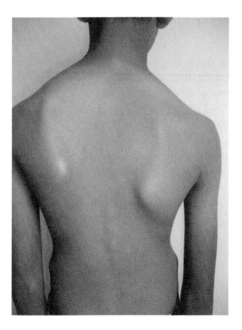

FIGURE 7.7A   A 16-year-old being followed up at the orthopedic department for his back pain was found to have scoliosis. He was tall and slim and had hyperextensible joints. He was referred to the dermatologist for a second opinion.

Based on the case description and Figure 7.7a, what are your differential diagnoses?

1. Marfan syndrome
2. Ehlers–Danlos syndrome (EDS)
3. Homocystinuria
4. Other fibrillinopathies

MARFAN SYNDROME

Diagnosis

Marfan syndrome

Discussion

Marfan syndrome is an autosomal dominant disorder of fibrillin-1 connective tissue with variable clinical manifestations, mainly affecting the cardiovascular, skeletal, and ocular systems. The patient is often, but not invariably, exceptionally tall, and the skeletal proportions are abnormal. The limbs are long, the excess being greatest distally, giving rise to arachnodactyly. Simple screening tests include:

1. The thumb sign (positive if the thumb when completely opposed in the clenched hand projects beyond the ulnar border)
2. The wrist sign (positive if the thumb and little finger overlap when wrapped around the opposite wrist)
3. The ratio of the lower segment (pubic ramus to floor) to the upper segment (height minus lower segment)

The skull is dolichocephalic, the paranasal sinuses are large, and the palate is high and arched. Other skeletal changes include hyperextensible joints, kyphoscoliosis, pectus excavatum, and flat foot.

The common ocular abnormalities include ectopia lentis (usually upward), a trembling iris (iridodonesis), myopia, and retinal detachment; less frequent are blue sclerae and heterochromia of the iris.

Aneurysmal dilatation of the ascending aorta is the most important abnormality of the cardiovascular system. Aortic dilatation may begin in childhood. Aortic and mitral incompetence are common with mitral valve prolapse occurring in 80% of cases (Burrows, 2016; Ellington & Francomano, 2023).

Cutaneous abnormalities are not uncommon: elastosis serpiginosa perforans, striae atrophicae, papyraceous scars, and skin hyperextensibility (Siriwardena, 2021).

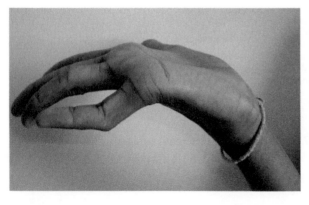 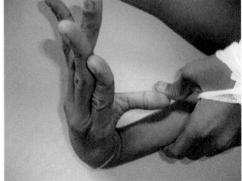

FIGURE 7.7B   (1) and (2) Hyperextensible joints in Marfan syndrome.

Investigations

This is a clinical diagnosis. Regular surveillance is required with imaging and monitoring of aortic root width and of the function of aortic and mitral valves.

Management

Aortic dissection is the most common cause of mortality; 50% of patients under 40 years old remain undiagnosed. With the introduction of β-blocking agents, angiotensin II receptor 1 blockers, and improvements in vascular and cardiac surgery, the prognosis has improved greatly and treated patients can have near-normal life expectancy.

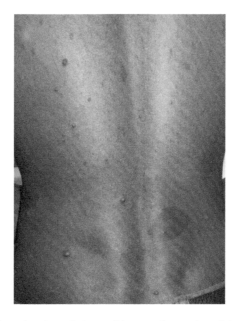

FIGURE 7.8   A 16-year-old boy developed these skin papules and nodules recently. He has had hyperpigmented birth marks since birth.

Based on the case description and Figure 7.8, what are your differential diagnoses?

1. Café-au-lait macules in neurofibromatosis
2. McCune–Albright syndrome

NEUROFIBROMATOSIS

Diagnosis

Neurofibromatosis 1 (NF1)

Discussion

NF1 is an inherited neuroectodermal abnormality, characterized by the presence of six or more café-au-lait macules (CALMs), axillary freckles, multiple neurofibromas, Lisch nodules (pigmented iris hamartomas), optic gliomas, and a first-degree relative. CALMs are the first feature of the disease to appear in all children. Skin-coloured neurofibromas appear late, starting in adolescence or early 20s.

Axillary freckling is pathognomonic (Crowe's sign) and appears later. Lisch nodules are asymptomatic but help to confirm the diagnosis. Kyphoscoliosis occurs in 2% of cases (Doser et al., 2022). The mode of inheritance is autosomal dominant, with almost 100% penetrance by the age of 5 years; 50% are due to gene mutations (chromosome 17 gene encodes a protein named neurofibromin), while incomplete or monosymptomatic forms are frequent (Irvine & Mellerio, 2016a).

Investigations

This is a clinical diagnosis.

Management

Symptomatic management only.

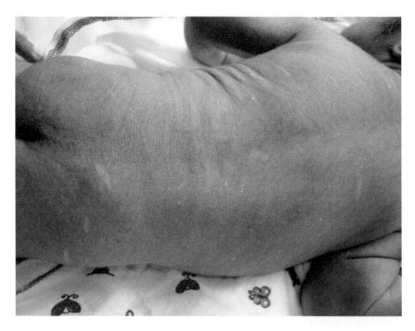

FIGURE 7.9 The neonatologist noticed multiple hypopigmented patches on the trunk and limbs in a newborn baby. This was an uneventful normal vaginal delivery. Radiological investigations detected cardiac and renal tumours.

Based on the case description and Figure 7.9, what are your differential diagnoses?

1. Ash-leaf macules in tuberous sclerosis complex
2. Congenital vitiligo

TUBEROUS SCLEROSIS COMPLEX

Diagnosis

Tuberous sclerosis complex

Discussion

Ash-leaf macules are easily visible in brown skin. Tuberous sclerosis complex was clinically suspected which was confirmed with radiological findings of associated cardiac rhabdomyomas.

Investigations

This is a clinical diagnosis. Radiological findings will help to establish the diagnosis.

Management

The parents were educated and the baby was monitored closely for neurological complications.

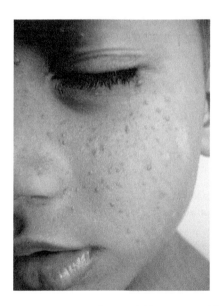

FIGURE 7.10A A 6-year-old boy came with acneiform eruption on the face for 3 months. He was on treatments for seizures. Careful examination revealed multiple hypopigmented patches on the face and the trunk.

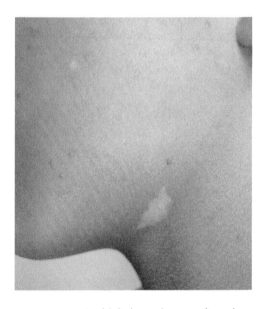

FIGURE 7.10B Multiple hypopigmented patches on the face (ash-leaf macules).

Based on the case description and Figures 7.10a and 7.10b what are your differential diagnoses?

1. Angiofibromas in tuberous sclerosis (adenoma sebaceum)
2. Plane warts

TUBEROUS SCLEROSIS COMPLEX

Diagnosis

Tuberous sclerosis complex (Same disease in an older boy)

Discussion

This is a genetic disorder of hamartoma formation in many organs, particularly the skin, brain, eyes, kidneys, and heart.

Skin lesions of four types are pathognomonic: "ash-leaf" white macules (abnormal melanocytes with reduced tyrosinase activity), angiofibromas (adenoma sebaceum), the shagreen patch (collagen tumour), and periungual fibromas. They may be seen in association with epilepsy and intellectual impairment.

White ovoid or ash-leaf-shaped macules, 1–3 cm in length, are a valuable physical sign because they may be found at birth or in early infancy. Angiofibromas usually appear between the ages of 3 and 10 years. They often become more extensive at puberty and then remain unchanged. The shagreen patch is an irregularly thickened, slightly elevated, soft, skin-coloured plaque, usually in the lumbosacral region. Periungual fibromas (Koenen tumours) appear at or after puberty as smooth, firm, flesh-coloured excrescences emerging from the nail folds. Other cutaneous manifestations include firm fibromatous plaques, especially on the forehead and scalp, soft pedunculated fibromas around the neck and axillae, and poliosis.

Cardiac rhabdomyomas, detected by echocardiography, occur in over 50% of infants. Renal involvement includes angiomyolipoma and renal cysts. Ocular signs occur in 50% of cases but may be hard to detect: retinal phacomas, pigmentary and other retinal abnormalities, scotomas or amaurosis, and hypopigmented spots in the iris (Słowińska et al., 2018).

Management

Management is symptomatic.

- Treat angiofibromas with a pulsed dye vascular laser.
- Papular/nodular lesions are best treated with a carbon dioxide laser.
- Neurosurgery should be considered when epilepsy is uncontrolled by drugs and/or focal lesion is detected (de Saint Martin et al., 2022).

REFERENCES

Bolton L (2022). New options to manage epidermolysis bullosa. *Wounds*;34(12):297–9.

Burrows N (2016). Genetic disorders of collagen, elastin and dermal matrix. In Christopher Griffiths, Jonathan B, Tanya B, Robert C, Daniel C, eds. *Rook's Textbook of Dermatology*, 9th edn. Hoboken: Wiley-Blackwell, 72.32p.

Chu DH, Jen MV, Yan AC (2016). Nutritional disorders affecting the skin. In Christopher G, Jonathan B, Tanya B, Robert C, Daniel C, eds. *Rook's Textbook of Dermatology*, 9th edn. Hoboken: Wiley-Blackwell, 63.25p.

Cook JC, Puckett Y (2022). Anetoderma (Jul 4). In *StatPearls* [Internet]. Treasure Island: StatPearls Publishing.

de Saint Martin A, Napuri S, Nguyen S (2022). Tuberous sclerosis complex and epilepsy in infancy: Prevention and early diagnosis. *Archives de Pédiatrie*;29(5S):5S8–13. doi: 10.1016/S0929-693X(22)00284-6.

Doser K, et al. (2022). Cohort profile: Life with neurofibromatosis 1—The Danish NF1 cohort. *BMJ Open* 20;12(9):e065340. doi: 10.1136/bmjopen-2022-065340.

Ellington M, Francomano CA (2023). Chiari I malformations and the heritable disorders of connective tissue. *Neurosurgery Clinics of North America*;34(1):61–5. doi: 10.1016/j.nec.2022.09.001.

Glutsch V, Hamm H, Goebeler M (2019). Zinc and skin: An update. *Journal Der Deutschen Dermatologischen Gesellschaft*;17(6):589–96. doi: 10.1111/ddg.13811. Epub 2019 Mar 15.

Gurevich I et al. (2022). In vivo topical gene therapy for recessive dystrophic epidermolysis bullosa: A phase 1 and 2 trial. *Nature Medicine*;28(4):780–8. doi: 10.1038/s41591-022-01737-y. Epub 2022 Mar 28.

Hamada T. (2002). Lipoid proteinosis. *Clinical and Experimental Dermatology*;27(8):624–9. doi: 10.1046/j.1365-2230.2002.01143.x.

Irvine AD, Mellerio JE (2016a). Hamartoneoplastic syndromes. In Christopher G, Jonathan B, Tanya B, Robert C, Daniel C, eds. *Rook's Textbook of Dermatology*, 9th edn. Hoboken: Wiley-Blackwell, 80.1p.

Irvine AD, Mellerio JE (2016b). Syndromes with premature ageing. In Christopher G, Jonathan B, Tanya B, Robert C, Daniel C, eds. *Rook's Textbook of Dermatology*, 9th edn. Hoboken: Wiley-Blackwell, 79.6p.

Itin P (2016). Ectodermal dysplasias. In Christopher G, Jonathan B, Tanya B, Robert C, Daniel C, eds. *Rook's Textbook of Dermatology*, 9th edn. Hoboken: Wiley-Blackwell, 67.12p.

Lovell CR (2016). Acquired disorders of dermal connective tissue. In Christopher G, Jonathan B, Tanya B, Robert C, Daniel C, eds. *Rook's Textbook of Dermatology*, 9th edn. Hoboken: Wiley-Blackwell, 96.20p.

McGrath JA (2016). Genetic blistering diseases. In Christopher G, Jonathan B, Tanya B, Robert C, Daniel C, eds. *Rook's Textbook of Dermatology*, 9th edn. Hoboken: Wiley-Blackwell, 71.1p.

Mohamed M, VoeT M, Gardeitchik T, Morava E (2014). Cutis laxa. *Advances in Experimental Medicine and Biology* 802:161–84. doi: 10.1007/978-94-007-7893-1_11.

Morris A (2016). Inherited metabolic diseases. In Christopher G, Jonathan B, Tanya B, Robert C, Daniel C, eds. *Rook's Textbook of Dermatology*, 9th edn. Hoboken: Wiley-Blackwell, 81.17p.

Searle T, Ali FR, Al-Niaimi F (2022). Zinc in dermatology. *The Journal of Dermatological Treatment*;33(5):2455–8. doi: 10.1080/09546634.2022.2062282.

Siriwardena C (2021). Disorders of connective tissue. In Ranawaka RR, Kannangara AP, Karawita A, eds. *Atlas of Dermatoses in Pigmented Skin*. Singapore: Springer, pp. 515–528. doi: 10.1007/978-981-15-5483-4_28.

Słowińska M, et al. (2018). Early diagnosis of tuberous sclerosis complex: A race against time. How to make the diagnosis before seizures? *The Orphanet Journal of Rare Diseases* 29;13(1):25. doi: 10.1186/s13023-018-0764-z.

Wright JT, Grange DK, Fete M (2022). Hypohidrotic ectodermal dysplasia. In Adam MP, Everman DB, Mirzaa GM, Pagon RA, Wallace SE, Bean LJH, Gripp KW, Amemiya A, eds. *GeneReviews®* [Internet]. Seattle: University of Washington, pp. 1993–2023.

Zou P, Du Y, Yang C, Cao Y (2023). Trace element zinc and skin disorders. *Frontiers in Medicine* (Lausanne) 17;9:1093868. doi: 10.3389/fmed.2022.1093868.

Skin Problems in Adolescence and Puberty in FST 5

8

Ranthilaka R. Gammanpila

INTRODUCTION

This chapter discusses skin problems in adolescence and puberty in brown skin (Fitzpatrick skin type V/ FST 5). These are discussed based on clinical photographs and easy-to-read question-and-answer format. Altogether this chapter discusses 13 clinical cases using 23 clinical photographs. Post-inflammatory hyper-and hypopigmentation is common and cosmetically concerned in darker skin.

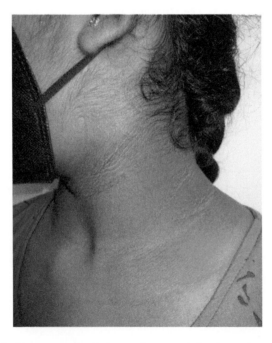

FIGURE 8.1 A 12-year-old girl presented with hyperpigmented discolouration of neck and axillary area for one year.

DOI: 10.1201/9781003321507-8

Based on the clinical history and Figure 8.1, what is your differential diagnosis?

1. Acanthosis nigricans
2. Ichthyosis vulgaris
3. Confluent and reticulated papillomatosis

ACANTHOSIS NIGRICANS

Diagnosis

Acanthosis nigricans

Discussion

Acanthosis nigricans is a velvety skin hyperpigmentation which occurs in association with diabetes mellitus, insulin resistance, hormone disorders (such as obesity, polycystic ovary disease, Cushing's, acromegaly, hypothyroidism, and Addison's diseases), medications like systemic glucocorticoids and oral contraceptives, and rarely, internal malignancies. Obesity is the commonest association. Clinically it is characterized by velvety skin darkening usually involving the intertriginous areas and skin folds including the back of the neck, axillae, and groin. Usually, the lesions have poorly defined borders and show skin thickening (Figure 8.13).

Investigations

This is a clinical diagnosis. Investigations are performed to identify associated diseases.

Management

It can fade over time by treating the causative factors (such as weight reduction). Keratolytics, such as topical retinoids, ammonium lactate, and topical vitamin D analogues, are used for its treatment. In severe cases, metformin and etretinate may be helpful.

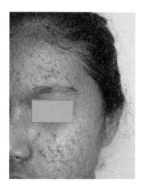

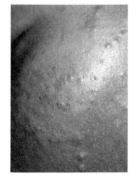

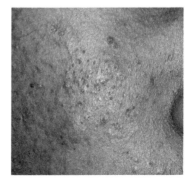

FIGURE 8.2A. A 12-year-old girl with papular eruption on the face.

FIGURE 8.2B Whiteheads (closed comedones). Note the oily skin.

FIGURE 8.2C Blackheads (open comedones).

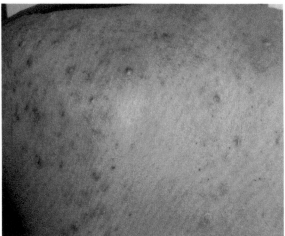

FIGURE 8.2D Truncal acne.

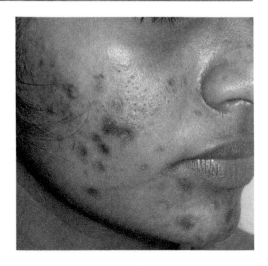

FIGURE 8.2E Post-inflammatory hyperpigmentation following acne.

Based on the case description and Figure 8.2a, what are your differential diagnoses?

1. Acne vulgaris
2. Acneiform eruption

ACNE VULGARIS

Diagnosis

Acne vulgaris

Discussion

Acne vulgaris is a chronic inflammatory disease of the pilosebaceous unit. The clinical lesions are non-inflammatory open (blackheads) and closed comedones (whiteheads) and/or inflammatory lesions: papules, pustules, cysts, and nodules. The face, back, and/or chest are the most frequently affected sites. This is the most common adolescent skin problem for which around 80% of teenagers seek treatments. In most, it is a transient disease of the teenage years. Post-inflammatory hyperpigmentation is commoner in darker skin (Fonseka, 2021a; Frazier et al., 2023).

Investigations

This is a clinical diagnosis.

Management

Management of acne depend on the severity and patients' expectations (Xu et al., 2021; Ludwig & von Stebut, 2023).

- *For mild to moderate acne*, first-line treatment options include a fixed combination of (a) topical adapalene with topical benzoyl peroxide, (b) topical tretinoin with topical clindamycin, or (c) topical benzoyl peroxide with topical clindamycin (Layton & Ravenscroft, 2023).
- *For moderate to severe acne*, first-line treatment options include (a) and (b) of the first point, and:
  - A fixed combination of topical adapalene with topical benzoyl peroxide, plus either oral lymecycline or oral doxycycline.
  - Topical azelaic acid plus either oral lymecycline or oral doxycycline.
- *For severe acne, cystic acne, or nodulo-cystic acne*, oral isotretinoin is the drug of choice.
- Topical or oral antibiotics should not be used as monotherapy or in combination with each other.

Review treatment response at 12 weeks; options that include an antibiotic (topical or oral) should be continued for more than 6 months only in exceptional circumstances.

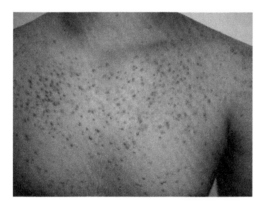

FIGURE 8.3   A 17-year-old boy came with this papular eruption on the front and back of the chest for one month.

Based on the case description and Figure 8.3, what are your differential diagnoses?

1. Acne vulgaris
2. Acneiform eruption
3. Steroid acne

ACNEIFORM ERUPTION/STEROID ACNE

Diagnosis

Acneiform eruption or steroid acne

Discussion

Monomorphic inflammatory lesions with an absence of comedones, often presenting acutely on sites not commonly affected by acne, should alert the diagnosis. The commonest cause in young females we observed was using skin-bleaching agents containing steroids (whitening creams). In young males, abuse of androgenic anabolic steroids, synthetic derivatives of testosterone and testosterone salts in the form of milk powders, or tablets are the commonest triggering factors. Corticosteroids may provoke an acneiform reaction regardless of their route of administration.

Investigations

This is a clinical diagnosis.

Management

Treatment is the same as in acne vulgaris. Find out the causative factors individually, and educate the patient on how they acquire the problem and to avoid triggering factors.

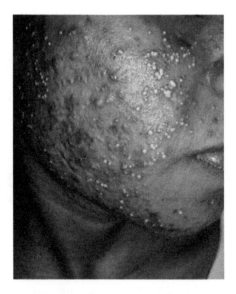

FIGURE 8.4   A 16-year-old girl came with worsening of acne while on oral doxycycline.

Based on the case description and Figure 8.4, what are your differential diagnoses?

1. Acne
2. Gram-negative folliculitis

GRAM-NEGATIVE FOLLICULITIS

Diagnosis

Gram-negative folliculitis

Discussion

Gram-negative folliculitis is due to overgrowth of Gram-negative organisms which can occur as a complication of long-term oral or, less frequently, topical antibiotic therapy used to treat acne. Sudden worsening of acne in spite of oral antibiotics should rouse the diagnosis. They present as eruption of multiple small follicular pustules or occasionally nodular lesions, most frequently localized around the perioral or perinasal skin. This results from overgrowth of Gram-negative organisms including *Klebsiella*, *Escherichia coli*, *Serratia marescens*, *Proteus mirabilis*, or *Pseudomonas aeruginosa* (Poli, 2012). These organisms replace the Gram-positive flora of the facial skin and mucous membranes.

Investigations

This is a clinical diagnosis.

Management

The current antibiotic should be discontinued, replacing it with either ampicillin (250 mg four times a day) or trimethoprim (600 mg/day) (Böni & Nehrhoff, 2003).

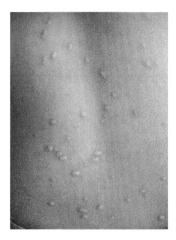

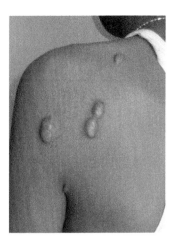

FIGURE 8.5A A 16-year-old girl requested curative treatments for these lesions that had developed a few months after generalized chickenpox infection.

FIGURE 8.5B Keloids on minor scratches in a 13-year-old boy.

Based on the case description and Figure 8.5a, what are your differential diagnoses?

1. Keloid
2. Hypertrophic scar

HYPERTROPHIC SCARS AND KELOIDS

Diagnosis

Keloid

Discussion

A **keloid** is a benign well-demarcated overgrowth of fibrotic tissue which extends beyond the original boundaries of a defect. A **hypertrophic scar** is similar, but remains confined to the original defect and tends to resolve after several months. Keloids and hypertrophic scars are cosmetically distressing, and often painful or pruritic.

Investigations

This is a clinical diagnosis.

Management

Non-essential surgery should be avoided in sites prone to keloids.

Despite numerous small case series advocating a wide range of therapies, there is no level-one evidence for any single treatment (Frech et al., 2023).

- Intralesional corticosteroids (most commonly triamcinolone acetonide) inhibit fibroblast proliferation and collagen synthesis. Injections may need to be repeated monthly and recurrence rates can be up to 50%.
- Pulsed dye and Nd:YAG lasers appear to be more effective, particularly in combination with intralesional corticosteroids or 5-FU.
- Surgical excision runs the risk of recurrence of an even bigger keloid. Intralesional (core) excision is preferable, and postsurgical intralesional steroids may prevent recurrence.

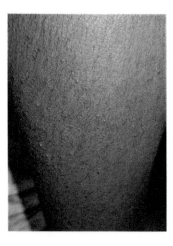

FIGURE 8.6 A 13-year-old girl is worried about these asymptomatic spiky lesions on her upper arms and thighs bilaterally.

Based on the case description and Figure 8.6, what are your differential diagnoses?

1. Lichen spinulosus
2. Keratosis pilaris
3. Follicular accentuation
4. Truncal acne
5. Atopic eczema

KERATOSIS PILARIS

Diagnosis

Keratosis pilaris

Discussion

Keratosis pilaris is an inherited abnormality of keratinization affecting the follicular orifices with varying degrees of keratotic follicular plugging, perifollicular erythema, and follicular atrophy. It is a very common condition affecting 50–80% of adolescents (Mehta & Ramam, 2023). KP starts in children, most commonly on the extensor surfaces of the upper arms, and can worsen around puberty. It can also appear on the thighs, buttocks, and lumbar area". Patients may complain about the "goosebump" or "chicken skin" appearance of their skin and rough texture. These small bumps can be skin-coloured, red, or brown. The skin can feel rough and dry, and can occasionally be itchy. Redness can also be found around many of the small bumps.

Clinical variants of KP: Keratosis pilaris may occasionally be associated with redness and pigmentation of the skin of the cheeks (*erythromelanosis follicularis facei et coli* and *keratosis pilaris rouge*), loss of eyebrow hair (*ulerythema ophryogenes*), small atrophic areas over the cheeks in late childhood (*atrophoderma vermiculatum*), and follicular atrophy and scarring alopecia in infancy (*keratosis follicularis spinulosa decalvans*) (Grullon et al., 2022).

Investigations

This is a clinical diagnosis.

Management

In the majority of patients KP is a mild cosmetic disorder which improves with age.

General Measures

Use of an exfoliating sponge or scrub in the shower or bath

Specific Measures

- Moisturizing cream that contains urea, salicylic acid, lactic acid, or alpha hydroxy acids (they either moisturize or help loosen the adherent scale in the follicles) is recommended.
- Topical retinoids can be used alone or combined with 10% urea-containing moisturizers.
- In severe KP, oral isotretinoin has been successful.
- Patients with severe fixed erythema from KP atrophicans faciei have been successfully treated with pulsed dye laser (Chu & Teixeira, 2016).
- Topical treatments—including Mineral Oil-Hydrophil Petrolat, tacrolimus, azelaic acid, and salicylic acid—are also effective at least for improving the appearance of KP. *(Maghfour et al., 2022, Suástegui-Rodríguez et al., 2022)*

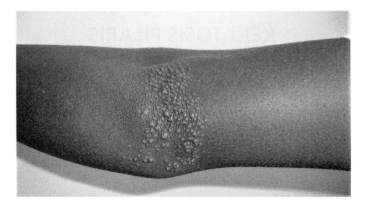

FIGURE 8.7   An 8-year-old boy came with these asymptomatic lesions on his elbows and knees bilaterally.

Based on the case description and Figure 8.7, what are your differential diagnoses?

1. Lichen spinulosus
2. Keratosis pilaris
3. Phrynoderma
4. Pityriasis rubra pilaris

LICHEN SPINULOSUS

Diagnosis

Lichen spinulosus or keratosis spinulosa

Discussion

Lichen spinulosus is a clinically distinctive variant of keratosis pilaris. LS generally erupts acutely and is asymptomatic. It is characterized by the appearance of hyperkeratotic follicular papules arranged into large plaques ranging from 2 to 5 cm in diameter. They are coarse to the touch. The patches are symmetrical and distributed on the trunk, buttocks, neck, knees, and elbows. The face, hands, and feet are usually spared. Plaques erupt in crops, grow rapidly, and then remain stationary. LS is a disease of children and young adults 16–26 years of age (Chu & Teixeira, 2016)

Phrynoderma, which literally means toad skin, is one of the cutaneous manifestations of vitamin A deficiency but may also be associated with other nutritional deficiencies. It manifests as follicular hyperkeratosis.

Investigations

This is a clinical diagnosis. Histological findings of lichen spinulosus are similar to those found in keratosis pilaris.

Management

There is no specific treatment for lichen spinulosus and in most cases it resolves spontaneously within 1–2 years, although it can persist for decades in some patients. The mainstays of treatment are topical retinoids and keratolytics.

Some patients may find the following useful (Bhoyrul & Sinclair, 2020):

- Non-soap cleansers (soap may exacerbate the dryness)
- Moisturizing cream applied twice daily
- Keratolytic agents including lactic acid (5–12%), salicylic acid (3–5%), and urea (10–20%)
- Topical retinoids, which are gels or creams available on prescription. For the first few weeks of treatment, redness and peeling of the treated areas can be expected. Topical retinoids should not be used in pregnancy.

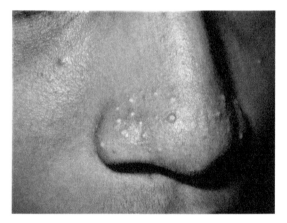 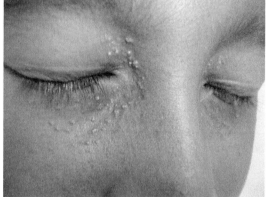

FIGURE 8.8A A 15-year-old girl came with these asymptomatic lumps on her nose and face for 6 months. On examination, multiple tiny yellowish translucent papules on the nose were noted.

FIGURE 8.8B Milia on the periorbital area in an 8-year-old boy.

Based on the case description and Figure 8.8a, what are your differential diagnoses?

1. Sebaceous adenoma
2. Acne
3. Trichoepithelioma
4. Milia/Milium

MILIUM/MILIA

Diagnosis

Milia

Discussion

Milia are isolated or grouped small uniform spherical white papules with a smooth non-umbilicated top. They are firm, white or yellowish, rarely more than 1 or 2 mm in diameter, and appear to be immediately beneath the epidermis. They are usually noticed only on the face, and occur in the areas of vellus hair follicles, on the cheeks and eyelids particularly. They feel soft and may release their gelatinous contents when punctured.

- *Clinical variants* (Lear & Madan, 2016)
- *Milia en plaque* appear as a cluster of milia on an erythematous, oedematous base. These are most commonly seen in the postauricular area.
- *Juvenile colloid milium* are multiple translucent yellowish papules on the cheeks, nose, and perioral skin; onset is usually before puberty. It is familial.

Investigations

This is a clinical diagnosis. Histopathology is performed in diagnostic difficulty; it shows colloid degeneration and the presence of colloid in dermal papillae.

Management

Incision of the overlying epidermis and expressing the contents is curative. Recurrence is uncommon. Spontaneous disappearance occurs in many milia in infants.

Laser ablation or puncturing the milia or electrodessication can be effective. Topical tretinoin may be effective.

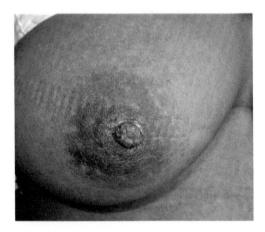

FIGURE 8.9   A 16-year-old teenager came with an itchy, oozing, eczematous rash on her nipple and areola.

Based on the case description and Figure 8.9, what are your differential diagnoses?

1. Nipple eczema
2. Irritant contact dermatitis
3. Allergic contact dermatitis
4. Paget's disease of the breast

NIPPLE ECZEMA

Diagnosis

Nipple eczema

Discussion

Eczema around the nipple and in the areola is not uncommon in young women. This is commoner in breastfeeding mothers, who are atopic. When it is bilateral, allergy to brassieres should be considered. If it does not respond to conventional treatments, and in cases of old age, Paget's disease of the breast should be considered which warrants skin biopsy. Eczema lacks the sharp, raised, and rounded margin and the superficial induration of Paget's disease (Reynaert et al., 2023).

Investigations

This is a clinical diagnosis.

Management

Mild topical steroids with frequent emollients would cure the disease. If it is bilateral look for possible allergens, such as black fabric dye and synthetic fabric materials in brassieres.

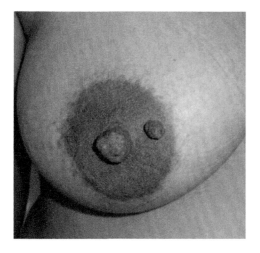

FIGURE 8.10A A 17-year-old girl wanted to get rid of this lump.

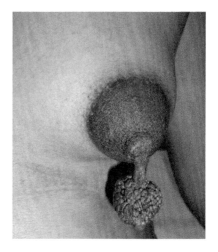

FIGURE 8.10B Pedunculated nipple papilloma.

Based on the clinical history and Figure 8.10a, what is your differential diagnosis?

1. Skin tag
2. Nipple papilloma
3. Breast carcinoma

NIPPLE PAPILLOMA

Diagnosis

Nipple papilloma

Discussion

Papillomas are common benign growths of cosmetic concern.

Investigations

This is a clinical diagnosis.

Management

Excision under local anaesthesia is curative.

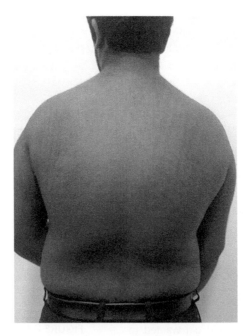

FIGURE 8.11   A 16-year-old obese boy presented with light-coloured (hypopigmented) horizontal bands on the back of his trunk for one year. (Photographed by Dr. Ajith P. Kannangara.)

Based on the clinical history and Figure 8.11, what is your differential diagnosis?

1. Physiological striae
2. Adolescent striae

OBESITY-RELATED SKIN PROBLEMS (PHYSIOLOGICAL STRIAE, SKIN TAGS)

Diagnosis

Physiological striae

Discussion

Striae, or stretch marks, are indented streaks that often affect the abdomen, buttocks, thighs, back, breasts, axillae, and groin. Striae are a form of dermal scarring associated with stretching of the dermis. They often result from a rapid change in weight (weight gain or weight loss) or are associated with endogenous or exogenous corticosteroids. Proposed mechanisms relate to hormones, physical stretch, and structural alterations of dermal collagen and elastic tissue. Striae are more common in females than in males and may be more common in certain races. They can appear more prominent in dark-skinned individuals. A positive family history is a risk factor for striae. The initial striae rubrae are slightly raised pink or violaceous linear marks (striae rubrae), which fade over months to years to hypopigmented, atrophic, wrinkled scars (striae albae). The marks are perpendicular to the direction of skin tension. They fade with time. In pregnancy, they occur on the abdomen, breasts, and thighs. In adolescents, they are common on thighs, buttocks, breasts (females), and back (males).

Investigations

This is a clinical diagnosis.

Management

Silicone gels are recommended for atrophic scars and may be used in striae distensae. Published results are difficult to interpret.

Tretinoin cream has been reported to be possibly useful in striae rubrae.

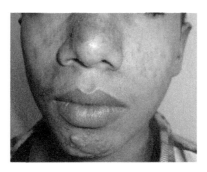

FIGURE 8.12 A 15-year-old boy with erythematous papular pustular eruption on the face for 6 months.

Based on the case description and Figure 8.12, what are your differential diagnoses?

1. Acne vulgaris
2. Rosacea

ROSACEA

Diagnosis

Rosacea

Discussion

Rosacea is a disorder that usually presents in middle age (peak onset between 35 and 50 years). It is a chronic disorder that primarily affects the face with a tendency to facial erythema and involving the eye. The cause of rosacea is unknown. Up to 25% of patients have a family history of the condition, indicating a significant genetic predisposition in some individuals. A common feature in the majority of patients is the presence of facial erythema. This boy has papulopustular rosacea that mimics acne vulgaris.

Patients present a spectrum of clinical features that differ according to each subtype (Fonseka, 2021b).

Erythematotelangiectatic Rosacea (ETTR) Patients with ETTR usually complain of a gradual increase in facial redness. This affects the central face but is not confined to this region, with the lateral cheeks, the ears, and sometimes the sides of the neck also being affected.

Papulopustular Rosacea (PPR) Patients with PPR give a history of developing groups of "spots, red bumps, or pimples" that are located principally on the proximal cheeks, central chin, nose, and central forehead. The presence of oily skin, open and closed comedones, cystic lesions, and scarring are features supporting the diagnosis of acne vulgaris.

Phymatous Rosacea (PR) Rhinophyma (the commonest form of PR and seen typically in male patients) may appear de novo (without preceding inflammatory changes) or occur in a patient with pre-existing PPR.

Ocular Rosacea (OR) Patients who develop OR frequently complain of a sensation of dryness with slight itch or a "gritty" feeling of the eyes in early-stage disease.

Investigations

This is a clinical diagnosis.

Management

Management differs according to the clinical type. Following are general measures for all the clinical types (Ludwig et al., 2023; Frank, 2016).

- Avoid undue sun exposure.
- Use sun-protective measures (apply daily sun block cream all year round and wear a hat) because chronic UV damage will contribute to facial erythema, especially in patients with ETTR. Physical sunscreens based on zinc or titanium are best tolerated.
- Many patients with rosacea have dry, easily irritated skin. Daily application of a moisturizing cream is important for such patients.
- Avoidance of potential irritants (abrasive soaps, astringents, perfumes, aftershave lotions, and skin-peeling preparations) is important because they tend to aggravate the facial erythema.

- Patients with a tendency to flushing (mainly those with ETTR) should avoid agents that provoke flushing such as hot drinks, spicy foods, alcohol and some drugs, and precipitating or exacerbating factors (e.g., stress, temperature).

Management of papulopustular rosacea. Sun avoidance, sun protection, moisturizing, and cosmetic cover should be undertaken as for ETTR. For active inflammatory lesions select a topical agent such as metronidazole 0.75% gel or cream, azelaic acid 15% gel, ivermectin 1% cream, or sodium sulfacetamide 10% and sulphur 5% preparations.

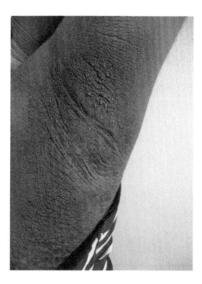

FIGURE 8.13 A 12-year-old obese girl presented with multiple warty lesions on axillae associated with blackish thick pigmented skin.

Based on the clinical history and Figure 8.13, what is your differential diagnosis?

1. Skin tags and acanthosis nigricans
2. Plane warts
3. Molluscum contagiosum

SKIN TAGS

Diagnosis

Skin tags

Discussion

A skin tag, also known as fibroepithelial polyp, soft fibroma, and acrochordon, is a benign skin lesion that affects about 50% of adults as well as obese children. Skin friction, obesity, and hormonal disturbances, especially diabetes mellitus, are the main risk factors. They are usually asymptomatic, soft, and skin-coloured. They may appear irritated and inflamed. Clinically, skin tags present in three clinical pictures including multiple small papules distributed on intertriginous areas like the neck and axillae, solitary or multiple soft filiform lesions anywhere on the body, and solitary large or giant soft fibromas on the genital area, especially on the penis and labia majora.

Investigations

Diagnosis is mostly clinical.

Management

Simple excision under local anesthesia. Electrocautery is preferred over cryotherapy, because of the increased risk for post-cryotherapy scarring.

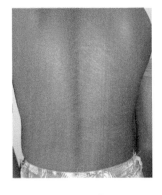

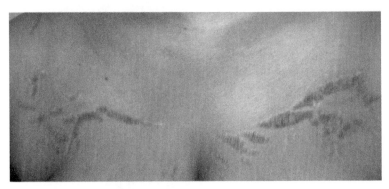

FIGURE 8.14A This 14-year-old boy's mother is worried about these asymptomatic skin lesions that have appeared over the last 6 months.

FIGURE 8.14B Steroid striae following topical application of clobetasol on the chest as a bleaching cream.

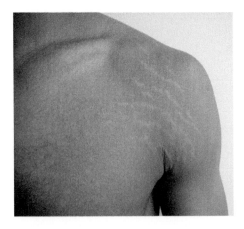

FIGURE 8.14C Striae in a 17-year-old boy who was doing bodybuilding exercises.

Based on the case description and Figure 8.14a, what are your differential diagnoses?

1. Adolescent striae
2. Steroid striae

ADOLESCENT STRIAE (PUBERTAL GROWTH STRIAE)

Diagnosis

Adolescent striae (pubertal growth striae)

Discussion

Striae (stretch marks) are visible linear scars which form in areas of dermal damage produced by stretching of the skin. They are characterized histologically by thinning of the overlying epidermis, with fine dermal collagen bundles arranged in straight lines parallel to the surface. Striae are associated with growth spurts, e.g., body-building or pregnancy; they may reflect structural abnormalities of connective tissue such as in Marfan syndrome or the effect of glucocorticoids (Borrelli et al., 2021).

Striae are often associated with growth spurts in adolescent males; they are normally all horizontally arranged right across the back (Elsedfy, 2020). Early lesions may be raised and irritable, but they soon become flat, smooth, and livid red. Their surface may be finely wrinkled. In darker skin the redness is not apparent and striae are generally paler than the surrounding skin. After some years, they fade and become inconspicuous.

Investigations

This is a clinical diagnosis.

Management

There is no proven treatment, but in the case of common adolescent striae, the patient may be reassured that in time they will become less conspicuous.

REFERENCES

Bhoyrul B, Sinclair R (2020). Successful treatment of keratosis follicularis spinulosa decalvans with an 800-nm diode laser. *Dermatologic Surgery*;46(6):849–50. doi: 10.1097/DSS.0000000000001892.

Böni R, Nehrhoff B (2003). Treatment of gram-negative folliculitis in patients with acne. *The American Journal of Clinical Dermatology* 4(4):273–6. doi: 10.2165/00128071-200304040-00005.

Borrelli MR, Griffin M, Ngaage LM, et al. (2021). Striae distensae: Scars without wounds. *Plastic and Reconstructive Surgery* 1;148(1):77–87. doi: 10.1097/PRS.0000000000008065.

Chu AC, Teixeira F (2016). Acquired disorders of epidermal keratinization. In Christopher G, Jonathan B, Tanya B, Robert C, Daniel C, eds. *Rook's Textbook of Dermatology*, 9th edn. Hoboken: Wiley-Blackwell, 87.11p.

Elsedfy H (2020). Striae distensae in adolescents: A mini review. *Acta Biomedical* 19;91(1):176–81. doi: 10.23750/abm.v91i1.9248.

Fonseka S (2021a). Acne. In Ranawaka RR, Kannangara AP, Karawita A, eds. *Atlas of Dermatoses in Pigmented Skin*. Singapore: Springer, pp. 503–510. doi: 10.1007/978-981-15-5483-4_26.

Fonseka S (2021b). Rosacea. In Ranawaka RR., Kannangara AP., Karawita, A, eds. *Atlas of Dermatoses in Pigmented Skin*. Singapore: Springer, pp. 511–4. doi: 10.1007/978-981-15-5483-4_27.

Frank CP (2016). Rosacea. In Christopher G, Jonathan B, Tanya B, Robert C, Daniel C, eds. *Rook's Textbook of Dermatology*, 9th edn. Hoboken: Wiley-Blackwell, 91.1p.

Frazier WT, Proddutur S, Swope K (2023). Common dermatologic conditions in skin of color. *American Family Physician (AFP)*;107(1):26–34.

Frech FS, Hernandez L, Urbonas R et al. (2023). Hypertrophic scars and keloids: Advances in treatment and review of established therapies. *The American Journal of Clinical Dermatology* 20. doi: 10.1007/s40257-022-00744-6.

Grullon K, Ashi SA, Shea CR, Ruiz de Luzuriaga AM, Stein SL, Rosenblatt AE (2022). Follicular keratosis of the face in pediatric patients of color. *Pediatric Dermatology*;39(2):231–5. doi:10.1111/pde.14946.

Layton AM, Ravenscroft J (2023). Adolescent acne vulgaris: Current and emerging treatments. *The Lancet Child & Adolescent Health*;7(2):136–44. doi: 10.1016/S2352-4642(22)00314-5

Lear JT, Madan V (2016). Cutaneous cysts. In Christopher G, Jonathan B, Tanya B, Robert C, Daniel C, eds. *Rook's Textbook of Dermatology*, 9th edn. Hoboken: Wiley-Blackwell, 134.4p.

Ludwig RJ, von Stebut E (2023). Entzündliche dermatosen auf pigmentierter haut [Inflammatory dermatoses in skin of color]. *Dermatologie* (Heidelb);74(2):84–9 (German). doi: 10.1007/s00105-022-05096-0. Epub 2023 Jan 2.

Maghfour J, Ly S, Haidari W, Taylor SL, Feldman SR (2022). Treatment of keratosis pilaris and its variants: A systematic review. *The Journal of Dermatological Treatment*;33(3):1231–42. doi: 10.1080/09546634.2020.1818678.

Mehta N, Ramam M (2023). Comment on "follicular keratosis of the face in pediatric patients of color". *Pediatric Dermatology*;40(1):222–3. doi: 10.1111/pde.15071. Epub 2022 Dec 5.

Poli F (2012). Differential diagnosis of facial acne on black skin. *The International Journal of Dermatology*;51 (Suppl 1):24–6, 27–9 (English, French). doi: 10.1111/j.1365-4632.2012.05559.x.

Reynaert V, Gutermuth J, Wollenberg A (2023). Nipple eczema: A systematic review and practical recommendations. *Journal of the European Academy of Dermatology and Venereology* 25. doi: 10.1111/jdv.18920.

Suástegui-Rodríguez I, Camacho-Rosas LH, Peralta-Pedrero ML, et al. (2022). Keratosis pilaris treatment: Evidence from intervention studies. *Skinmed* 31;20(4):258–71.

Xu J, Mavranezouli I, Kuznetsov L et al. (2021). Guideline committee. Management of acne vulgaris: Summary of NICE guidance. *BMJ* 20;374:n1800. doi: 10.1136/bmj.n1800.

Index

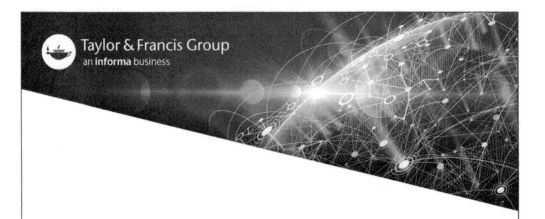
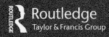
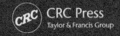

Printed and bound by CPI Group (UK) Ltd, Croydon, CR0 4YY

17/10/2024

01775663-0010